T0321594

Pursuing the Elixir of Life

Chinese Medicine for Health

Pursuing the Elixir of Life

Chinese Medicine for Health

Hong Hai MD, PhD
Karen Wee BSc(Hons), BMed

Nanyang Technological University and The Renhai Clinic, Singapore

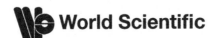 World Scientific

NEW JERSEY · LONDON · SINGAPORE · BEIJING · SHANGHAI · HONG KONG · TAIPEI · CHENNAI · TOKYO

Published by

World Scientific Publishing Co. Pte. Ltd.

5 Toh Tuck Link, Singapore 596224

USA office: 27 Warren Street, Suite 401-402, Hackensack, NJ 07601

UK office: 57 Shelton Street, Covent Garden, London WC2H 9HE

Library of Congress Cataloging-in-Publication Data
Names: Hong, Hai, 1943–   author. | Wee, Karen, author.
Title: Pursuing the elixir of life : Chinese medicine for health / by Hong Hai and Karen Wee.
Description: New Jersey : World Scientific, 2016. |
    Includes bibliographical references and index.
Identifiers: LCCN 2016047614| ISBN 9789813207035 (hardcover : alk. paper) |
    ISBN 9789813207042 (pbk. : alk. paper)
Subjects: | MESH: Medicine, Chinese Traditional | Acupuncture Therapy
Classification: LCC RM184.5 | NLM WB 55.C4 | DDC 615.8/92--dc23
LC record available at https://lccn.loc.gov/2016047614

British Library Cataloguing-in-Publication Data
A catalogue record for this book is available from the British Library.

Printed in Singapore

Preface

The title of the book reflects the perennial hope of Man to find the Elixir of Life that confers on him longevity if not also immortality. Immortality remains a distant dream, even though high-powered biomedical scientists believe they are getting close to understanding why we age and look to the prospect of quantum leaps in life extension.

For the humbler Chinese physicians, the elixir of life is the practice of life cultivation or *yangsheng* that enables us to live in good health up to the natural limit of the human lifespan, declared by the ancient medical classic the *Huangdi Neijing* to be around a hundred years. The main theme of this book revolves around *yangsheng*. We hope it will enable the reader to take the first step toward achieving health and longevity.

This book has been compiled from lectures to many batches of participants in courses run by the authors over the years. It sets out in plain language what we have found to be a difficult subject to teach in English, not only because many terms in Chinese medicine do not translate well into other languages, but also on account of the concepts and ideas in Chinese medicine being deeply intertwined with culture and philosophy. Nevertheless, the continuing good attendance of our courses encourages us in the conviction that no subject, however difficult, cannot be explained in simple terms if the instructor has thought deeply about it and teaches it with a passion.

We begin the book with a few introductory chapters on the principles of Chinese medicine before delving into the secrets of health cultivation and longevity.

As this is an introductory book, no attempt has been made to define terms in a rigorous manner that would satisfy the Chinese medical scholar. Instead we have taken liberties to explain the subject in such a manner that a person who a basic knowledge of science can relate to its concepts and methods and make use of them in daily living.

This book can be read together with its companion volume *Principles of Chinese Medicine: A Modern Interpretation* (Imperial College Press) by Hong Hai, which treats the theory of Chinese medicine in greater depth and discusses the scientific and philosophical aspects of Chinese medicine. We would like to thank Imperial College Press for permission to adapt some materials from that volume for use in this book. We are also grateful to our editor Ms Joy Quek for her meticulous and tireless effort bringing out the book.

Hong Hai
Karen Wee
30th September 2016

Contents

1

From Spirits to Natural Science

The origins of Chinese medicine

Glamorous Hong Kong Phoenix TV hostess Liu Hairuo was seriously injured in a British train accident in May 2003, suffering severe multiple fractures to her ribs and damage to her head, liver, lungs and spine. She underwent several surgeries at the Royal Free Hospital in London but remained in a coma on life-support. British doctors conjectured she was brain dead and were prepared to pull the plug and end her life.

Her grieving family refused to give up and decided to seek an alternative in Chinese medicine. A month after the accident she was admitted to Beijing's Xuanwu Hospital. An astonishing miracle happened. After receiving treatment with a combination of Chinese and Western medicines, Liu Hairuo regained consciousness, made a full recovery and resumed her career, with the additional mission of speaking and writing about her experience of Chinese medicine snatching her from the gates of death.

One of the key medications used to treat Liu was the humble Angong Bezoar or *angong niuhuang wan* (安宫牛黄丸), a common traditional resuscitative medication used to revive patients who faint from excessive stress or exposure to heat, also often used in Chinese hospitals for patients in the immediate aftermath of a stroke.

In the SARS world epidemic in 2002, the average mortality rate was 12–25% in countries outside China, compared to an estimated 7% in China where a combination of Chinese herbal medications and Western drugs were used.[1]

There are numerous impressive anecdotes of the power of Chinese medicine to cure unusual illnesses, as well as millions of patients throughout the world who seek and find Chinese medical cures for both acute and chronic illnesses. Such accounts give comfort to Chinese physicians and their patients. Their belief in the efficacy and scientific nature of Chinese medicine is frequently challenged by Western medical practitioners, who may be uninformed about Chinese medicine and therefore view it with scepticism over its safety and efficacy.

In fairness and to be more convincing, Chinese physicians need to view the successful results of Chinese therapy with

[1] Report of the International Expert Meeting to review and analyse clinical reports on combination treatment for SARS (2004) referenced in http://apps. who.int/medicinedocs/en/d/Js6170e/3.html (retrieved 8 September 2016).

caution as most of their methods have not been subjected to clinical trials to validate that such results can be repeated with some consistency. This is the reason why large resources throughout the world are now being allocated to tests using modern methods of evidence-based medicine.

Nevertheless the weight of historical evidence found in numerous case records suggests that there is something special in Chinese medicine, despite its ancient origins and its lack of use of modern technology, that makes it worth our while to try to understand it better and be more discerning as to when to use it for our health and for healing our illnesses.

In 2014 the Cleveland Clinic, which together with the Mayo Clinic rank as the most renowned in the United States, started a TCM section offering acupuncture and herbal medicinal treatments to the public, despite its acknowledgment that much of TCM treatments has not undergone clinical trials expected of medical interventions in the US. This far-sighted decision indicates the clinic's willingness to try therapies that are wanted by patients, many of whom feel better after receiving such treatment and prefer them to conventional Western medicine. It speaks for the perceived potential that Chinese medicine can offer mankind in health care from its thousands of years of accumulated experience and wisdom.

1.1 Chinese Medicine in Antiquity

What is Chinese medicine and how did it begin?

Chinese medicine has origins going back thousands of years when herbalists like the legendary Shen Nong (circa 2500 BC) painstakingly combed the hills and forests of China to seek out leaves, roots and animal parts that had healing powers. The early practitioners of acupuncture used sharpened stones to exert pressure on selected points in the body and discovered that this could ease pain and promote flows in the body to achieve internal balance and healing. This laid the foundation of the complex science of acupuncture, now practised in modern clinics throughout the world and approved for health insurance claims in America.

But was Chinese medicine always based on science? For thousands of years, a large part of it was not. In ancient China, healing was often attributed to pacifying the spirits as it was believed that people fell ill because they were possessed by evil spirits and demons. Mediums had to be employed to pray and appease or drive away these spirits. There were similar practices in ancient Korea where Shaman priests were employed. Greece and Rome in antiquity practised 'Temple Medicine' by which sick people would spend nights sleeping in temples in the belief that in their dreams the Gods would appear to deal with the spirits that troubled them.

It was only about two thousand years ago during the great flourishing of carefully recorded medical cases by the great physicians of the Han dynasty (206 BC–220 AD) that the collective wisdom and experience of these physicians were captured and compiled in the greatest of all Chinese medical classics, the *Huangdi Neijing* (黄帝内经) (*The Yellow Emperor's Canon of Medicine*). This monumental work marked the beginning of the scientific Chinese medicine.

The *Neijing* declared that illnesses were not caused by spiritual agents but by natural forces, which are basically climatic, dietary, lifestyle and emotional in nature. Over the next 2000 years, hundreds of legendary physicians further developed these ideas into the Chinese medicine taught today in medical colleges and practised in clinics all over the world.

TCM is thus the product of a long history of experimentation, conjectures about the inner workings of the body, and the equivalent of thousands of clinical trials in which different herbal and acupuncture formulations were tried on generations of patients. These results were painstakingly recorded in case studies of eminent physicians. Even in modern societies today, these case studies continue to lend important insights into the methods and ideas of these physicians.

1.2 Chinese Medicine Modernises

Up to the first half of the 20th century, Chinese medicine was mainstream medicine, but its position was increasingly challenged by scholars who had studied Western medicine abroad. On the 5th of May 1919, an event of historic importance happened that later became known as the "May 4th Movement" (五四运动). Students at Peking University, tired of a weak China, once the most powerful and technologically advanced nation in the world being humiliated by foreign military incursions in her territories, marched and protested against unfair treaties imposed by foreigners.

The May 4th Movement was in fact the beginning of the modernisation of China. Returned scholars were determined to change China by introducing science and technology, and a greater measure of public participation in governance. One of the consequences of this movement was that the scientific nature of Chinese medicine came into question, as there were differences in the science as practised in ancient China and that in the West. Attempts were made by Western-educated physicians to reject Chinese medicine altogether and replace it with Western medicine. Several decades of debate and contention followed, and the issue was not settled until the ascendancy of Chairman Mao Zedong following the 1949 Chinese Revolution.

Mao was a believer of Chinese medicine, calling it a "a treasure trove of Chinese wisdom" but had no illusions that it had exclusive or complete knowledge of the science of health and healing. He felt Chinese medicine had to be modernised by absorbing some of the ideas and methods of Western medicine, in particular carefully recording and systematising medical knowledge into textbooks similar to those used in Western medical schools. As a result of Mao's intervention, Chinese medicine was preserved in China and its teaching modernised through new textbooks written in contemporary plain language. Medical education was carried out through new colleges of Chinese medicine offering undergraduate and post-graduate degrees. Chinese medicine taught formally and practised this way became known as 'Traditional Chinese Medicine' (TCM). In China and Taiwan today, Chinese and Western medicine are practised side by side in many major hospitals and clinics. In many ways, their patients enjoy the best of both worlds

It should be noted that TCM as taught and practised under government regulatory supervision is different from a variety of old Chinese practices not incorporated in modern textbooks. These comprise mainly what we may call folk medicine which uses methods and ideas that do not fall within mainstream of Chinese medicine. TCM is the form of Chinese medicine which governments in China, Hong Kong, Taiwan, Malaysian and Singapore recognize and license physicians to practice.

2

Why Chinese Medicine Matters

Ten distinguishing characteristics of TCM

What is special about Chinese medicine that makes it a mystery to sceptical Western observers yet passionately embraced by myriads of users in the Orient? Why does it enjoy a sizable and growing following in Europe, Australia and America?

Chinese medical thought and practice represent the synthesis of its ancient culture and philosophy with the clinical experience of generations of physicians dedicated to conquering illness and promoting health. Many of the ideas in TCM may be found in Chinese literature and ancient philosophical writings. Hence Chinese medicine is not just a method of healing, but a culture of living a full life through enjoying good health and finding fulfilment in harmony with nature and society.

Several distinguishing features of TCM make it different from Western medicine. These include the holistic character of TCM and its emphasis on harmony. This in turn leads to seeking treatment for the root of a health disorder rather than symptomatic relief.

TCM is patient-centric in the sense that treatment is customised to the patient, so that two patients with the same disease may receive quite different medications because their underlying conditions and body constitutions may be different. A chronic headache often treated with an analgesic like paracetamol in Western medicine would be diagnosed by a Chinese physician as having arisen from one of several root causes, among which might be weakness of vital energy known as *qi*, internal heat arising from over-consumption of rich foods, or an accumulation of phlegm within the body that disturbs the mind. For each condition, a different treatment is prescribed by TCM.

The Chinese physician takes into account the inherent constitution of the patient, which affects what kind of medication his body is likely to find congenial. Little wonder then that Chinese physicians have a lot of time for the iconoclastic eminent Oxford professor of medicine William Osler who famously said that "The good physician treats the disease; the great physician treats the patient who has the disease."[2]

On the important issue of what causes disease, we shall see that TCM takes quite a different view from Western etiology, and

---

[2]William Osler Quotes. http://www.brainyquote.com/quotes/authors/w/william_osler.html (retrieved 8 September 2016).

that the treatment modalities and methods are consequently different and special to TCM.

Let's take a look at ten aspects of TCM that make it special and different from conventional biomedicine.

2.1 Holism

The concept of holism is central to Chinese medical philosophy. Holism, as the term implies, means viewing things as a whole rather than in parts. It requires seeing the big picture and regarding the body as a functioning organism with all its parts working together in harmony and in accordance with regularities in nature.

In his celebrated verse about the majestic Mount Lu in Jiangxi province, the renowned poet Su Dongbo (苏东坡) declared, "I do not know the true face of Lushan, but only because I am in the midst of the mountain." ("不知庐山真面目, 只缘身在此山中.") When you are inside the mountain, you can only see the foliage, tree trunks, green undergrowth, insects and wild animals, but you have no idea what the whole mountain actually looks like. To view the mountain as a whole, you have to stand away from it at a distance. You can also then better understand the environmental influences that shape its ecology.

A similar idea carries through to Chinese medicine. If we only look at a portion of the body that is unwell, for example the stomach that is suffering pain, but do not observe other important signs that the body manifests, like lassitude and aversion to cold that may be related to the stomach disorder, we can only have an incomplete understanding of the illness. And if we only peer at the cells and genes that are the building blocks of the body, what chance is there that we understand the workings of the body as a whole?

Focusing on blood, cells, genes and hormonal secretions, as is the mainstay of biomedicine, may well deprive us of an understanding of the bigger picture. Of course, Western medicine also looks at the body as a whole. However because of the dominance of advanced technology allowing us to observe disease at the microscopic level, an approach that is usually termed as 'reductionist medicine', there is a tendency to place insufficient emphasis on the holistic approach. It is well known in medical circles that the average Western physician spends more time looking at laboratory reports and test data on the computer screen, and less time talking to his patient, than his Chinese counterpart.[3] Albert Einstein in his later years noted that scientists were becoming too reductionist and neglecting holism when he lamented, "Many scientists...seem to be like somebody who has seen thousands of trees but has never seen a forest."

Two thousand years ago when the *Huangdi Neijing* was compiled, physicians did not have microscopes and laboratories to look at cells and analyse blood and body fluids, hence they could not be reductionist even if they wanted to be so. They could only look at the body's external manifestations. Hence Chinese diagnosis and therapies focussed on looking at the body as a whole and sought explanations for illnesses accordingly. This naturally has severe limitations, which we should take into account in using Chinese medicine to treat disease.

The combination of Chinese holism and biomedical reductionism would be the ideal approach to medicine. Unfortunately, this has many challenging issues, yet to be resolved in most countries, although patients can on their own consult both

---

[3] See for example, Evans, D (2005) *Placebo: The Belief Effect.* Oxford: Harper Collins.

Chinese and Western physicians and sometimes succeed in using both selectively to achieve optimal results. We shall have more to say on this subject in the closing chapter of the book when we conjecture the convergence of Chinese and Western medicine in the distant future.

2.2 Flow, Balance and Harmony

The Chinese understanding of health revolves around smooth flow of *qi*, blood and other fluids, as well as internal balance and harmony of *yin* and *yang*.

We have yet in this book to define and explain terms like *qi*, *yin* and *yang,* although most readers would already have a nodding acquaintance with them. New readers of Chinese medical books usually have this initial difficulty. It is the chicken and egg problem: to explain principles, you need to have the basic concepts; but the concepts are empty without principles to which to relate them. For such new readers, we request your patience as the concepts will be explained in the next two chapters of the book. After you have read those, you may return to this chapter for a deeper understanding.

Flow in Chinese medicine means *qi*, blood and other fluid flows in our body. Lack of flow is associated with pain, hence the aphorism "When there is no flow, there is pain; when there is no pain, there is flow" (不通则痛, 不痛则通). This means that the source of pain is poor flow. For example, if we have the pain in a joint, it could be because *qi* and blood are not flowing well around the joint area. Indeed, *qi* stagnation, blood stasis, dampness, phlegm are all related to impeded flows, and are the basic causes of many illnesses.

Consider the common condition of joint pain known as arthritis. Chinese medicine looks at it in terms of imbalance that causes *qi* or blood not to flow properly, resulting in inflammation as wear and tear in the body is not repaired and cleared up properly. Chinese medicine would relate the underlying cause of the arthritic pain to blockages of *qi* and blood. From the Western medical perspective, explanations may be sought in dysfunctioning microscopic components of the blood and the immune system. To treat arthritic pain, Chinese medicine would promote flow of blood and *qi* to reduce the impediments that underlie inflammation rather than use painkillers or anti-inflammatory drugs like steroids that provide symptomatic relief.

The absence of flow is stagnation. The legendary physician, Hua Tuo observed that "a door that is opened regularly will not have sticky hinges." If we do not at least periodically open and close a door, it will develop sticky hinges that may eventually seize up. For health, every part of the body must be functioning, flowing or moving. In modern parlance, we "use it or lose it."

The importance of balance and flow for health can be illustrated with two further examples:

(1) Stress can cause liver *qi* to stagnate; resulting in digestive problems, insomnia, foul moods. The appropriate therapy is to restore *qi* flow.

(2) Weakness of kidney *yin*, which can be caused by exposure to heat, is a form of imbalance in which *yang* dominates as a result of weakened *yin*. The person feels warm, vexatious and thirsty, and sweats excessively. Therapy aims to nourish *yin* to restore balance.

With smooth flows and balance, harmony is achieved in the body. Internal harmony means the *yin* and *yang* forces are balanced within the body whereas external harmony means the cycles of nature are not violated and there is harmony between us and nature. At night, our body enters the *yin* cycle and we should calm down and prepare for sleep. But if we decide to go to the gym and have a workout, we are violating the natural order and some may not be able to sleep well after that. Even if we do get to sleep readily, the internal working hours of our body may be adversely affected in the long run. In other words, our body was evolved in nature to sleep at night and not be subjected to mental or physical stress as we enter the evening hours and progress into the night. Violating this amounts to disharmony with nature's cycles. In general, healthy living requires harmony between us and the forces of nature.

2.3 Deficiency and Excess

Another important concept in Chinese medicine is that of 'deficiency' (*xu* 虚), also known as asthenia, which refers to the body being lacking in certain substances or energies such as *qi*, blood, *yin* and *yang*. The antithesis of deficiency is 'excess' (*shi* 实), also known as sthenia, which implies that our bodies have certain things in excess, such as too much heat or an excessive level of *yin* or *yang*. Deficiency and excess must both be absent in order for the body to be balanced. For example, if the body is subjected to too much dryness or heat, this can damage *yin* and the body may develop deficiency of *yin*, which is manifested in such symptoms as dryness of throat and internal heat.

2.4 Syndromes

Another key concept in TCM that distinguishes it from Western medicine is its emphasis on the differentiation of 'syndromes'. A syndrome (*zheng* 证) is a collection of symptoms that form an identifiable pattern. A very common syndrome is 'heat', which must be understood differently from our normal concept of heat that causes substances to feel hot to touch; it is also different from excessive body heat that results in a high temperature as when one is having a fever. When we have a TCM heat syndrome (and the body is said to be 'heaty'), it means that we have symptoms like a dry throat, a feeling of vexatiousness, and we manifest a yellow coating (fur) on the tongue; the pulse is a faster than normal. The body temperature may be normal, or it may be elevated, but having a temperature is not a necessary part of having heat in the TCM sense.

Further on this book, we shall come across many other syndromes, like dampness, or deficiency of kidney *yin*, and understand how TCM deals with them to restore balance and health in your body. These syndromes form the core conditions diagnosed by TCM methods. Every condition of illness is treated according to the syndrome or syndromes from which the body suffers.

TCM therapy consists mainly of identifying syndromes that indicate underlying imbalances and disharmonies in the body, and treatment consists of resolving these syndromes. More importantly, preventing illness consists of detecting syndromes in their early stages and resolving them before they become clinically identifiable diseases.

2.5 TCM is Patient-Centric

In view of its emphasis on differentiating and treating syndromes, TCM can be regarded as being 'patient-centric' rather than 'disease-centric'. This means that for the same disease, there may be different underlying syndromes, and treatment should be according to the syndromes present, and these may vary from one person to another. For example, the treatment for chronic constipation for patient A is to moisturize the large intestine which means to produce more fluids as the stools are too dry. The underlying syndrome for patient A is *yin* deficiency, which is accompanied by internal heat and dryness. In the case of patient B, the constipation may be caused by poor peristalsis movement, as a result of which one has difficulty pushing out stools from the colon. The underlying syndrome is this case is *qi* deficiency which weakens the peristaltic movements. Such conditions are common in the elderly whose *qi* weaken with age. The remedy is to strengthen *qi* with a suitable *qi* tonic.

In the above cases, we see that the same condition (disease) of constipation is treated differently for two persons according to the underlying syndrome for each person. Hence, there is a saying in TCM: "Different treatment for the same disease; and same treatment for different diseases" (同病異治, 異病同治). This principle and the foregoing examples illustrate the underlying meaning of TCM being patient-centric: it focuses on the syndrome of the individual patient, and not on finding a common cure for constipation that can be used for all patients. Professor Osler would have approved.

2.6 Emphasis on Preventing Illness

In Chinese medicine, the highest attainment of a physician is to treat the illness that has not happened yet (治未病). This requires the skill of the physician in identifying a patient's syndromes in their early stages before it develops into clinical illness.

For example, a person with *yin* deficiency of the lung may show mild deficiency heat symptoms like a dry throat and vex-axiousnes, with a red tongue and little fur. If left untreated, he could develop a persistent dry cough that is hard to heal. The physician must nip the problem in the bud while it is still evolving and relatively easy to treat.

This explains why in ancient China a family physician is rewarded with a better bonus each year if he has dispensed very little medicine during the year to treat illnesses. He has prevented mild syndromes from developing into diseases that require strong medication, but instead used diet, herbal tonics and other mild prophylactic concoctions, and inculcated good living habits in the family, to prevent serious conditions from developing.

2.7 Food as Medicine

In Chinese medicine, food and medicine are from the same source (药食同源). In other words, there is no firm distinction between food and medicine. Many of the herbs that we come across in this book are added to food and form part of cooked recipes. Most of the common foods that we eat, if used correctly, can also serve as medicine. Chinese medicine emphasizes the strong relationship and lack of distinction between food and medicine.

In fact, whenever possible, it is better to treat ourselves with common everyday foods rather than medicinal herbs.

2.8 Causes and Treatment of Illnesses

In Western medicine, many diseases are traced to viral agents, bacteria, malfunction of cells, hormonal imbalance and the like, viewing the body largely at the microscopic level. The approach to treatment of disease is to destroy germs that are troubling the body; if there is hormonal imbalance, as with low estrogen or testosterone levels, as can occur in menopausal women and ageing men respectively, a popular biomedical treatment is to use hormonal therapy, introducing hormone supplements to the body. If your red blood cells count is low, a blood transfusion or taking iron pills to supplement the haemoglobin in the red blood cells are the usual options. This kind of intervention reduces diseases to the cellular level, hence is commonly termed as reductionist.

In contrast, Chinese medicine looks at illnesses in terms of internal imbalance or impeded flows, and the treatment is always to restore balance and flows. In this sense, it is considered more holistic.

Is there a way to reconcile the Western and Chinese approaches? Essentially, they represent alternative ways of looking at the functions of the body, leading to different approaches to therapy. It would be improper and somewhat narrow-minded to claim that one approach is right and the other wrong. What matters is that the treatments be effective.

One of the biggest questions in medicine has always been: what is the cause of disease and illness? That may sound very simple, but it really is not. Take for example the common cold. I recall some years ago, I caught a cold and I mentioned it to a virologist that I caught the cold because I suffered a chill after exercise, having exposed myself to cold air conditioning while hot and sweating. He disagreed violently and said the cause of my cold was the common cold virus, known as the rhinovirus. The virus can be found anywhere in the air. I asked him why I had the cold and he had not. My learned scientist friend started to waver, and said it might be because I had been working too hard and not getting enough sleep, and my immune system was weakened.

So was it the virus that caused the cold or my weakened immune system that succumbed to the chill in the airconditioned room? The virus is not something that we can control to prevent colds. What we can control are our habits and lifestyles, such as looking after our bodies and avoiding exposure to chills, and getting enough sleep to keep our immune system from being weakened. From the TCM perspective, the real cause of the cold was the chill invading a weakened body defence system (known in TCM as *'zheng qi'* 正气).

It should now be obvious that causation is not such a straightforward matter. Many factors are involved, sometimes called causal factors or risk factors. What really matters for practical purposes is which factors we can control and manipulate to prevent disease; for practical purposes, these can legitimately make claim to being causes.

As a broad generalisation, Western medicine, or biomedicine, can be said to be more focused on immediate or proximate causes, whereas TCM views illness as disharmonies at a more basic level.

2.9 TCM Treatment Modalities

Chinese medicine has basically 4 modes of therapy. The oldest of these is acupuncture and moxibustion, which occupies a separate major section of *The Yellow Emperor's Canon of Medicine*. There is an erroneous but popular belief that acupuncture is used only to treat pain. In TCM practice, it is used for a wide variety of conditions, such as irritable bowel syndrome, gynaecological problems, erectile dysfunction, insomnia, and depression. In fact for every condition treatable with medication, there is an equivalent intervention using acupuncture. Experienced physicians make the judgment of whether to use acupuncture or medication, or both in combination.

A related mode of therapy is moxibustion, performed by burning the moxa herb (*aiye*艾叶) and placing it near the desired acupoint or part of the body so as to provide a warming action to the body. Such a mode of therapy is especially useful for treating cold syndromes.

The most common treatment modality is the use of herbal medicines. These herbs can come in many different forms, the most common being parts of a plants like the chrysanthemum flower or wolfberry seeds, but they can also be in the form of insects and animals like the silkworm or centipede, or the horn of a deer, or minerals like oyster shells. These different forms of medicine are formally called Chinese *material medica* (中药). For convenience in this book we refer to all of them as 'herbs'. Each herb has its own therapeutic action and the physician usually prescribes them based on the syndromes present in the patient.

The third method of therapy is *qigong*, which involves breathing and meditation techniques. Practiced correctly with professional instruction, it can be very helpful in the treatment of many illnesses. The main aims of *qigong* are to improve the flow of *qi* and blood in our bodies, and restore *yin* and *yang* harmony.

Tuina is also considered a mode of therapy in Chinese medicine. It works in a similar manner to acupuncture, following the same principles of working the meridians and acupoints. Instead of using needles to trigger the therapeutic action of the acupoints, hand and finger pressure is applied on the acupoints and meridians to help to restore balance and flow in the body. Child *tuina* is usually performed on children up to five years of age, particularly those who are averse to acupuncture.

2.10 Philosophy and Science in TCM

TCM is basically an empirical science based on observations of the human body. The popular Chinese term 实事求是 which means "Seek truth from the facts" is the core of the Chinese philosophy in medicine. It de-emphasises ideology and rejects biases based on long-held beliefs, but instead enjoins people to look at the facts and derive truth from them. Former Chinese leader Deng Xiao Ping immortalised this ideology during a state visit to the United States when he declared that "it does not matter if the cat is black or white as long as it can catch mice." If it works, it is the truth, and we do not need not agonise or feel perplexed about the abstruse ideology or profound science behind it.

Over thousands of years, Chinese physicians experimented with different methods of diagnosis and therapy. For example, they found that certain herbal combinations worked for specific conditions, and patients got well after using them. They thought deeply about these experiences and developed a narrative of why their methods worked. This narrative eventually became working models and guidelines for diagnosis and therapy, and now forms the main body of Chinese medical theory. It is a practical and pragmatic approach to medicine.

Much of the numerous case records and anecdotes collectively form a body of clinical evidence for the efficacy of these diagnostic and therapeutic models. To be sure, such evidence does not have the same level of statistical rigour as the randomised clinical trials of modern evidence-based medicine applied to mass-produced modern pharmaceuticals. There is indeed a good case for encouraging TCM researchers to conduct more clinical trials based on larger and controlled samples of patients. It has also been pointed out that controlled clinical trials can evaluate the intervention or the herbal product, but not the full human experience that occurs when traditional medicine is delivered by trusted practitioners in its 'cultural home'.[4]

---

[4] Director General of the World Health Organisation Dr Margaret Chan has suggested that clinical trials on alternative medicine like TCM should take into account its complex interaction with patients because of its deep social

This is a complex subject and the reader who is interested in this subject can find a full account of it in a companion volume to this book.[5]

Chinese medicine has a long history of experimentation. Shen Nong recorded the therapeutic effects of hundreds of herbs by tasting them himself. Centuries later, Li Shi Zhen (李时珍) (1518–1539 AD) compiled *Bencao Gangmu* (本草纲目) from extensive medical case records. Experimentation is the most fundamental basic form of science. TCM as an experimental science is not of the same genre or rigour as physics or biomedical science. While much remains to be done to strengthen its claims with more extensive and rigorous clinical trials, there is a great deal of it that we can use safely and with a high chance that they help us to achieve health and fight disease.

---

and cultural origins: "The scientific method was not designed to accurately evaluate the full human experience that occurs when traditional medicine is delivered by skilled, experienced, and trusted practitioners in its cultural and historical home. Controlled clinical trials can evaluate the intervention or the herbal product, but not the full experience." http://who.int/dg/speeches/2015/traditional-medicine/en/ (retrieved 12 September 2016).

[5] Hong, H (2016) *Principles of Chinese Medicine: A Modern Interpretation.* London: Imperial College Press.

3

The Precious Ingredients of Life

Basic substances in the body

In Chinese medical theory, the body contains the fundamental ingredients of *qi*, blood, and *jing* (collectively known as the three precious ingredients or *sanbao* 三宝) as well as body fluids known as *jinye* 津液.

3.1 *Qi* (气)

In ancient Chinese cosmology, *qi* was regarded as the most basic constituent of the universe, the origin of all substances, processes and vital energy forces. Because of these ancient

Chinese beliefs, over time the word '*qi*' was adopted in many aspects of the Chinese language, and in modern times we find this word used in numerous daily concepts involving flow, movement, or energy. For example, *qixiang* (气象) means weather, *qizhi* (气质) refers to the innate quality of a person and *qise* (气色) the glow of health.

In Chinese medical theory, *qi* has a special meaning and should not be confused with its numerous applications in everyday language. In Chinese medical usage, *qi* has two aspects: it is a kind of vital force driving flow and change in the body, and it can be a kind of substance that stores the energy of the vital force. For example, *zongqi* (宗气) refers to the pectoral *qi* that according to ancient understanding resides below the sternum, akin to a reservoir of special energy that allows one to have a sonorous voice. A good singer would be regarded as having good *zongqi*. As a practical matter, in modern biological terms, when someone has a strong *zongqi*, we mean his lung and diaphragm muscles are strong, his respiratory tracts are clear, and his vocal cords in good condition. Thus having good *zongqi* is a way of saying one has this capability.

This example illustrates the importance for our understanding of Chinese medicine to regard medical terms like *qi* as denoting a certain capability and not necessarily any identifiable substance with measurable properties. Likewise, as we shall see later in this chapter, the concept of a pathogen like dampness does not refer to high humidity but a pathological condition which makes a person feel lethargic and experience digestive discomfort. We hope the reader keeps this point constantly in mind when reading books and articles on TCM, as it is a common source of confusion and perplexity when the reader cannot relate a TCM term to his understanding of the term in daily non-medical usage.

The meaning of *qi* in medicine would thus vary with context, depending on the part of the body or the body condition we refer to. In general, any physiological activity has some kind of '*qi*' behind it. Depending on the context *qi* could be a form of a vital force or stored energy in the organs essential to maintaining life activities, driving the functions of the viscera and meridians. Thus we speak of spleen *qi*, kidney *qi*, heart *qi* and other forms of *qi* that are involved in the functions of these organs.

Kinds and Sources of Qi

Qi can also be classified by its particular role in the body as a whole. Thus *weiqi* (卫气) is defensive armour at the outer layers of the body which prevents the invasion of pathogens; *yingqi* (营气) is a nutrient *qi* that circulates and nourishes the body; *Qi* in the lower abdomen area prevents prolapse of the lower organs, and *qi* in the skin prevents excessive sweating.

From where does the body get its *qi*? The acquisition of *qi* comes in two stages. Through our parents, we are born with some *qi* known as 'congenital *qi*' or *yuanqi* (元气) stored in the kidney. The amount of congenital *qi* inherited from parents affects the health and development of the baby. After birth, we acquire more *qi* from food and exercise; air from breathing and blood are also involved in the production of *qi*. The spleen, which governs digestion, transforms food into nutrients; with the assistance of the liver, nutrients are transformed to *qi*.

3.2 Blood (血)

In TCM, blood (*xue*) has a wider meaning although its definition is similar to blood in modern physiology. Blood has the functions of nourishing and moistening the body, transporting turbid *qi* for excretion and fuelling mental activities and sound sleep. Our minds require sufficient blood to carry out normal activities. If a person is deficient in blood, he may suffer from insomnia, poor concentration and forgetfulness, as blood is inadequate for nourishing his mind for mental work as well as sound sleep.

The circulation of blood is propelled by the heart and driven in the body by *qi*. *Qi* and blood are like inseparable twins and share a close relationship which is described as "*Qi* is the marshal of blood and blood is the mother of *qi*." (气为血之帅, 血为气之母).

Qi is the marshal of blood because *qi* promotes the flow of blood. Without *qi* as the driving force, the flow of blood is stagnant and it cannot be transported to all parts of the body. Furthermore, *qi* participates in the production of blood, and also helps to keep blood within the blood vessels, preventing it from leaking out. Therefore, when a person is *qi*-deficient, he may also be vulnerable to bleeding as he does not have enough *qi* to hold the blood within the blood vessels.

Blood is said to be the mother of *qi* because it produces and carries *qi*. When *qi* accompanies blood, it moves along correct paths without being dispersed. This explains why when someone suffers from severe haemorrhage there is a loss of not only blood but also *qi*.

Thus it can be seen that blood and *qi* are like two sides of a coin, interdependent on each other, in some respects like *yin* and *yang*. Based on their characteristics and functions, *qi* is *yang* in nature and blood is *yin* because *qi* is like a driving force, constantly moving and pushing all the body activities and warming up the body whereas blood does the quiet but equally important job of nourishing and moistening the body.

3.3 Body Fluids (津液)

Another important entity in our body is the body fluids *jinye* (津液). We know in practice there are hundreds of kinds of body fluids in our body such as hormonal secretions and digestive juices. But in the Chinese model, all these fluids are classified under *jinye*. The scope of *jinye* is thus very wide and covers many functions of the various body fluids and secretions found in modern physiology.

Like *qi* and blood, *jinye* is produced from food by the organs. The thin body fluids are usually found in muscles, skin and orifices whereas the thick body fluids are found in the organs and marrow. Its main functions are to nourish, participate in blood production and transport turbid *qi*.

3.4 Jing (精)

The body also has a more mysterious substance known as essence or *jing* (精). *Jing* is stored in the kidney and inherited from one's parents. *Jing* is *yin* in nature and carries with it the inherited characteristics of the parents. From a biomedical perspective, *jing* is like the genes that a child is endowed with, carrying the genetic characteristics of both parents.

Jing is closely related to *qi*. Besides carrying the endowment of parents' characteristics, *jing* is also a source of *qi*, as it can be converted to *qi*. Likewise, *qi* can be used to replenish *jing*. If we regard *qi* as a form of energy, *jing* is the stored form of energy like fuel.

A special form of *jing* is the male semen. Semen contains sperms that carry the characteristics of the father that are passed on to the child. Hence it is important for the human body to have sufficient *qi* to replenish *jing* and enable the reproductive process.

The relationship between *qi* and *jing* is so close that one sometimes refers to them as one entity, *jingqi* (精气). There are many other interesting aspects of *jing* but we shall not cover them in this introductory volume, and the reader is encouraged to read more advanced texts to understand *jing* further.

4

The Inner Workings of the Human Body

A unique narrative drawn from experience

Chinese medicine has an understanding of the workings of the human body that originally was influenced by ancient philosophy and cosmology. The ancients believed that the inner universe within the body was a sort of replica (microcosm) of the outer universe, hence they looked to certain regularities observed in nature and tried to see similar patterns within the human body. In practice, physicians had to contend with the realities of human illness and sought models of the workings of the human body that would guide them to heal the sick. The result was a set of principles designed to best fit their clinical experience, refined over hundreds of years into a narrative behind a system of medicine that has stood the test of time.

We describe below two of the fundamental models of the human body's inner workings: the *Yin-Yang* Principle and the Five-Element Model. Although historically derived from ancient cosmology, in medicine they are empirically-based models for practical use and no longer have any cosmological or spiritual implications. We shall touch on the scientific rationale for these models, but a more thorough treatment is outside the scope of this book and must be left to a more advanced text.[6] In this chapter we explain how these models work, and the intriguing ways they help in medical diagnosis and therapy.

4.1 The *Yin-Yang* Principle

The idea of *yin* and *yang* is fundamental to the Chinese conceptual framework. It draws on observations of nature where things tend to exist in pairs — male and female, soft and hard, night and day — and that there are relationships and interactions between these two contrasting entities that capture the profound essence of harmony and balance, not just in the natural world but also in human and societal relationships. So influential has been the notions of *yin* and *yang* that they are a regular part of the lexicon of Western writers and long ago had made their way into the Oxford Dictionary.

Yet *yin* and *yang* as a fundamental principle in medicine takes on a mystique that puts Chinese medicine in a dim light

---

[6]For example, Chapter 6 of Hong (see footnote 5).

for those uninitiated in the subtleties of Chinese medical thought. Only after having studied Chinese medicine and grasped the deep influence that this principle exerts on how human health is understood does one begin to appreciate its intrinsic beauty and elegance.

These concepts originated many thousands of years ago, even before the time of the *The Book of Changes*, commonly referred to as the *I-Ching* (易经) of the Western Zhou dynasty (circa 1000–750 BC). The *I-Ching* has detailed treatment of *yin-yang* and contains numerous conjectures of its implications for human living. Taoist philosophy drew inspiration from the *I-Ching* and used it in for divination and religious purposes.

However, a thousand years later, when the concept of *yin* and *yang* was applied to Chinese medicine in the Han dynasty, it took on secular characteristics. By the time of the *Huangdi Neijing*, the *yin-yang* principle as applied to medicine had become a practical model for understanding relationships in nature, with no spiritual or religious significance.

In the concept of *yin* and *yang*, the world is one ruled by dualism. As the founder of Taoist philosophy *Laozi* explained, if there is no darkness there can be no light. How can we explain darkness except as the absence of light? *Yin* and *yang* therefore cannot exist without each other.

Consider the concept of beauty. Beauty does not have much meaning unless we have something ugly with which to contrast it. If you think that this is just common sense and represents no great insights, you are probably right. But there exist other notions of existence of beauty. Students of Greek philosophy will note that the *yin-yang* line of thinking differs from that found in the classic *The Republic* by Plato, arguably the greatest Western philosopher of all times. Plato conceived of a world of absolutes like beauty, justice, and love to which he gave the term 'forms'. Forms have existence in their own right, independent of contrasting entities like ugliness or injustice.

We shall not delve further into these philosophical arguments here. Suffice it to say that the Chinese have always been a pragmatic people. They tend to see both sides of a condition or of an argument, the *yin* and the *yang* aspects, and seek harmony through a balance of both. Indeed it can be said that the ruling passion of Chinese culture has been the search for harmony, which is why the Chinese word for harmony *he* (和) is found in so many compound words in Chinese vocabulary, almost invariably to imply a desired or satisfactory state of affairs.

Male and female characteristics are often used as examples for illustrating the nature of *yin* and *yang*. Apart from the biological differences between male and female, some characteristic of *yang* tend to be found more in the stereotyped male: physically strong, unyielding, transparent, analytical, and insensitive. The characteristics of *yin* which are mellow, yielding, unfathomable, discursive and sensitive, not surprisingly are associated with the stereotyped female (Table 4.1).

Some of these characteristics carry through to Chinese medicine. For example *qi* embodies energy and movement and is *yang* in character; blood which runs deep and quietly nourishes the body is *yin*. An overly warm body has a predominance of *yang*; conversely a overly-cool body has an excess of *yin*. We shall find many more such examples as we navigate through the complexities of TCM thinking in the book. The sense of what is *yin* and what constitutes *yang* will gradually sink into your psyche so that you learn to recognise them readily when you encounter them. You will find a similar experience with TCM concepts such as dampness, wind and phlegm. By exposure to and working with these concepts, understanding will gradually percolate into your system of thought.

Table 4.1 *Yin* and *Yang* characteristics

Yang 阳	**Yin** 阴
Male	Female
Light	Darkness
External	Internal
Day	Night
Strong	Mellow
Rigid & Unyielding	Flexible & Yielding
Hard	Soft
Transparent	Unfathomable
Hot, Dry	Cool, Moist
Fast, Hurried	Slow, Patient
Analytical	Discursive
Insensitive	Sensitive

4.1.1 *Guide to the application of the Yin and Yang principle*

1. Mutual opposition and support. One of the principles of *yin* and *yang* is that they have mutual opposition, that is, they oppose and restrain each other. If we observe the symbol of *yin* and *yang* in Fig. 4.1, we notice that the dark portion *yin* exercises a restraining influence on the white portion representing *yang*.

2. The interdependence principle of *yin* and *yang* emphasises that they depend on each other for survival. Notice from the picture that each wraps around and supports the other, and one could not exist without the other. This intriguing situation in which two forces oppose but are also dependent on each other is one of the deep insights of Chinese philosophy. It may sound paradoxical, but that is much the

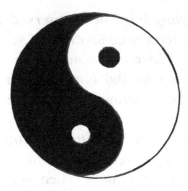

Fig. 4.1 Symbol of *yin* and *yang*

way the universe and life inside are structured. Somebody who opposes and restrains you is also somebody on whom you may be dependent.

When we apply this idea to behaviour in human society, we begin to understand better why Chinese philosophy emphasises balance so much. Chinese philosophy mostly does not indulge in absolutes, such as taking a cultural chauvinistic view that only one system of conduct or governance is correct. For example, it is entirely consistent with Chinese culture that socialism should exist side by side with capitalism and that a balance between them be struck for the healthy functioning of the economy.

In the human body, both the *yin* and *yang* forces have to be kept in balance. As in a human organisation, you need both the highly analytical, transparent and forceful persons among its leaders but you also need the softer and more flexible ones who are more forgiving of errors and allow deviation from the rules. This is because if you are driving the organisation with only pure *yang*-characteristic people, the organisation may eventually fail without the *yin* forces

to mellow the *yang*. It has been observed that in the historical rivalry between the civilisations of Athens and Sparta in
ancient Greece, Sparta became overly *yang* in nature,
run by oligarchs who did not believe in democracy and
emphasized military training for its citizens. It eventually
perished.

3.   The third principle is that *yin* and *yang* wax and wane.
     They rise and fall in cycles. There will be times that *yang*
     is dominant and other times when *yin* is dominant. The
     most obvious example that comes to mind is the day and
     night cycle. In Chinese medicine, we treat *yang* to be day
     and *yin* to be night. At 6 am when the sun is rising, *yang*
     is just starting to rise and by noon *yang* is at the peak.
     After noon, *yang* starts to weaken and by 6 pm *yang* has
     mellowed and *yin* comes in and starts to rise at 6 pm reach-
     ing a peak at midnight. After that it starts to decline and by
     6am the next morning, it has bottomed and *yang* resurges.

     This has implications for good living habits. We should
     rest and sleep at the *yin* part of the cycle and be active and
     doing things at the *yang* part of the cycle. This is because
     yang is strong during the day and we feel energetic for
     work. We should not be doing work at night but rather pre-
     pare for sleep early so that by midnight when *yin* is at the
     peak, we would be soundly asleep and the body is recuper-
     ating from the toils of the *yang*-dominated day. The best
     time to exercise is early in the morning when our body
     yang is rising.

     The *yin-yang* cycle can also be applied to the four sea-
     sons. Summer is when *yang* is at the maximum and starts to
     decline in autumn whereas the *yin* cycle is rising. By winter,
     yin is at its peak and when spring comes, *yang* is back and
     rising again.

4.1.2 *Yin-Yang imbalance*

There are many variations of *yin-yang* imbalance which causes the body to fall ill. Let's look at two common examples.

In example 1 (Fig. 4.2), when *yang* is in excess (which could be due to excessive ingestion of 'heaty' food or tonics), it generates excess heat whereas *yin* stays at the normal level. The manifestations of this condition may include fever, sore throat, a red tongue and fast pulse. The condition is termed excess heat (*shire* 实热); the treatment is to clear or dispel the excess heat using heat-clearing herbs such as the chrysanthemum flower.

In example 2 (Fig. 4.3) which is very common in hot climates, *yang* is at a normal level but *yin* has been damaged or weakened from overworking, exposure to hot weather and excessive sweating. As a result there is a deficiency of *yin*. By comparison with the deficient *yin*, *yang* has become relatively strong. In this condition, heat is also produced, known as deficiency

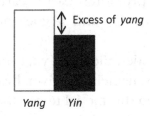

Fig. 4.2   Example 1

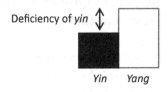

Fig. 4.3   Example 2

heat (*xure* 虚热) because the heat comes not from excessive *yang* but rather from the weakened or deficient *yin*. Women in the menopausal stage tend to have this condition and would usually present symptoms such as hot flashes, night sweating and dry skin. The remedy is not to expel heat, but rather to nourish *yin* using herbs that can help to strengthen *yin*, like wolfberry seeds and lily bulb.

4.2 The Five-Element Model

Another important TCM principle is *wuxing* (五行), usually translated as the Five Elements, but also sometimes called the Five Phases. *Wuxing* has origins in ancient cosmology where the world was considered to be made up of 5 elements: wood, water, fire, earth and metal. They were deemed to have certain interactive relationships with one another.[7]

One relationship is called inter-promotion which uses the analogy of "mother promotes (generates) child." Wood promotes fire, fire promotes earth, earth promotes metal and metal promotes water, and it goes on in that direction in a cycle (Fig. 4.4).

The ancients identified five vital solid organs known as the *zang* (脏) organs, namely the liver, heart, spleen, lung and kidney and borrowed this model to put them in an analogous combination (Fig. 4.5). They discovered from clinical experience that it fitted the way they perceived certain relationships among these organs, and therefore was helpful as a guide for the diagnosis and treatment of illnesses in these organs.

---

[7] Needham records some of the historical development of the five-element model in cosmology, pointing out that it had origins in and applications to relationship between the emperor and his ministers in ancient Chinese courts. See Needham, J (2016) *Science and Civilisation in China*, Vol VI, Part VI. Cambridge University Press.

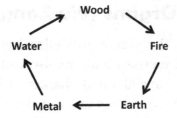

Fig. 4.4. The five elements

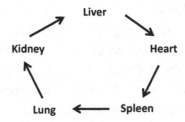

Fig. 4.5. The five *zang* organs

How should we understand the scientific basis for such a relationship among the organs of the body? On this subject, there are differences among Chinese medical thinkers. Orthodox scholars regard the five-element model as some kind of immutable law of nature akin to laws in physics. A more pragmatic view is to regard this as a model that roughly captures the experience of physicians observing relationships among organs in their clinical work. After experimenting with different combinations, this model was found to fit many of their observations and therefore became a good guide to their understanding of organ relationships. In science, this is called a *heuristic* model, discovered by experimentation to be helpful in explaining many observations. Hence the five-element model has become a useful tool for Chinese physicians in diagnosis and therapy. More will be said about this in Chapter 5 on diagnosis and therapies.

4.3 The Five Organs (Wu Zang)

In modern anatomy, the organs are defined as tissues that carry out related sets of functions and are also called 'somatic structures', that is, they have defined shapes and locations in the body. However, in TCM organs are not the same as organs in modern anatomy. Each organ is not a physical structure with a fixed location, but instead is a kind of conceptual representation of a set of physiological functions that feature in TCM diagnosis and treatment methods.

For example, the 'spleen' (*pi* 脾) in TCM represents functions related to digestion, hence when TCM talks of the spleen, it is talking principally about the equivalent of the digestive system. Likewise, the 'kidney' (*shen* 肾) in TCM represents not just the urine excretion function, but also growth, reproduction, marrow and brain functions, and the role of warming the organs. Thus the *shen* in TCM has a wide range of important functions, and is entirely different from the kidney as understood in modern anatomy and physiology.

This difference between the TCM organ and that in Western medicine is extremely important. Failure to recognise it leads to a great deal of confusion among laymen as well as incredulity among scientists uninitiated in Chinese medicine, who cannot accept an organ in TCM having such different functions from those they understand in modern physiology.

In Chinese Medicine, organs in general comprise not only the *zang* organs, for also the *fu* (腑) organs hence the term '*zang-fu*'. Each *fu* organ is paired with a *zang* organ that functions closely with it. The *fu* organs comprise the gall bladder, small intestine, stomach, large intestine and the bladder, paired with the liver, heart, spleen, lung and kidney respectively. The *zang* organs are considered solid and their main function is to produce and store essential substances such as *qi*, blood and essence which are vital for the daily activities of the body; on the other hand, the *fu* organs are hollow and mostly involved in the transportation and transformation of substances in the body that flow through them.

For example, the kidney (*shen*) stores essence which is necessary for the growth and development of the body besides processing urine, whereas the bladder (*pang guang* 膀胱) stores urine that needs to be excreted from the body.

There is a sixth *fu* organ, namely the trunk of the body, also known as the "triple burner" or *sanjiao* (三焦). The triple burner stretches from the thorax to the abdomen, and it is divided into three sections: the upper, middle and the lower. In Chinese medicine, based on the location of the *zang* and *fu* organs, the upper trunk contains the lung and the heart, the middle trunk contains the spleen, stomach, liver and gall bladder, and the lower trunk holds the kidney, bladder, small and large intestine. The main function of the triple burner is to act as the channel for *qi* and water transport.

4.3.1 *Functions of the zang organs*

Spleen

The spleen plays the role of the digestive system. It governs transportation and transformation of food, absorbing nutrients and transforming them into *qi* and blood for the vital body activities. The spleen is also known as the post-natal basis of life (后天之本) because it is the source of our *qi* and blood that are made from nutrition. After birth, our bodies constantly require *qi* and blood to grow and function. When we say someone has spleen-*qi* deficiency or 脾气虚, it means that the spleen is unable to absorb and transport the nutrients properly. As a result, the person will present symptoms such as poor appetite, lethargy, loose stools or a bloated stomach.

The spleen is said to 'command' blood, which refers to its role in helping to keep blood in the blood vessels and preventing it from leaking out, which results in bleeding. In TCM theory, some cases of internal bleeding can be attributed to spleen-*qi* deficiency.

Lung

The lung governs respiratory *qi* as well as production and circulation of *qi* in the whole body. Respiratory *qi* refers to the *qi* that we breathe in and out through our respiratory system. The lung also regulates the water passage for circulation and excretion purposes. The *Huangdi Neijing* makes the interesting observation that the lung is situated at the upper trunk of the triple burner, which is the highest point of the water passage and thus it can divert water to other parts of the body.

Kidney

The kidney is regarded as one of the most important organs in Chinese medicine. It is also known as the prenatal base of life (先天之本) as it stores essence *jing* which governs growth, development, reproduction and ageing. Essence increases as we grow hair and teeth start to form, and puberty sets in, reaching a peak at the physical prime age of our twenties and thirties, when our bodies are strongest and full of energy. As we pass our prime age, essence starts to decline and we develop white hair, loose teeth, and poorer complexion; andropause for men and menopause for women set in.

When we say that there is kidney deficiency in a child, this usually refers to having a low level of essence from birth, resulting in slow growth, poor hair and teeth development, and a smaller build. In the case of adults who have kidney deficiency, the symptoms are usually manifested in the reproductive system. Males may experience erectile dysfunction, and females possibly earlier onset of menopause.

Another function of kidney is to govern water metabolism which includes the excretion of urine, and in this narrow respect it is similar to the kidney in Western medicine.

The kidney is said to 'receive *qi*' in the sense that it helps the lung to govern respiratory *qi*. As the kidney is located at the lower trunk of the body, it helps to receive *qi* that is inhaled from the lung. Weakness in this function can be seen in patients who experience breathlessness, especially among the elderly, due to a decrease in kidney *qi*.

The kidney has a warming and nourishing function for internal organs. It produces and nourishes marrow which includes the spinal cord and brain marrow other than the bone marrow.

Liver

The liver has the function of dredging and regulating, which means it helps to ensure that the pathway of *qi* is smooth. Healthy *qi* flow can also lead to good blood flow, which will in turn help to promote circulation of blood and metabolism, assist the stomach in digestion and regulate mental activity. The liver also stores blood and helps to regulate the blood flow during menstruation.

Heart

One of the functions of the heart in Chinese medicine is to propel blood and participate in production of blood to nourish the body. The heart also governs mental activities through nourishing blood and *yin* of the heart. If a person has deficiency in heart blood, he would often experience problems such as

Table 4.2 Organ functions

Zang-organs	Functions
Spleen	• Governs transportation and transformation of food • "Commands" blood (keeps blood within vessels)
Lung	• Governs ("dominates") respiratory qi as well as production and circulation of qi in the whole body • Regulates water passage
Kidney	• Governs growth, development, reproduction & ageing • Governs metabolism of water including urine excretion • Receptions of qi (helps the lung govern qi) • Nourishes and warm the internal organs • Produces marrow
Liver	Dredges and regulates qi i.e. ensure its smooth flow in the body (*shuxie* 疏泄), and stores blood: • promotes circulation of blood and metabolism, assists the stomach in digestion, regulate mental activity through smooth flow of qi and blood • regulates menstruation through proper blood flow to the uterus
Heart	• Propels blood and participates in production of blood • Controls mind and governs mental activities

insomnia, poor memory, and difficulty in concentrating as there is insufficient blood to nourish the mind.

4.3.2 Applying the five-element model to the zang organs

Figure 4.5 earlier showed the correspondence between the five elements and the *zang* organs. TCM theory has some analogies that are useful as an aid to our remembering the relationship of the organ to a principal function.

For example, the kidney governs water metabolism and this explains why kidney is assigned to the water element. The heart pumps blood that warms the body, hence it is assigned to the fire element. The spleen governs 'transportation and transformation' of food into nutrients so that sufficient *qi* and blood are produced to sustain the body's metabolism. By analogy, the earth produces nutrients for the growth of the plants, hence the spleen is assigned to the earth element. The liver has the function of ensuring smooth *qi* flow and dislikes restriction, hence it is assigned to the wood element which has the property of growing from a sapling to a tall tree. The lung governs respiratory *qi* which has the property of purifying. This property is similar to that of metals, some of which have the ability to purify.

Application to Therapy

These five-element model is also applied in TCM therapy. A common application is to tonify the mother to strengthen the child (虚者补其母), which is indicated by the inter-promotion relationship between the elements. In other words, the health of the unborn child is dependent on the mother and the kind of nutrition she provides the child. This analogy is found to be useful in TCM therapy. For example, in the treatment of cough with phlegm, most physicians would not only treat the lung to clear the phlegm but also the spleen (its mother). The spleen in TCM is thus also regarded as a source of phlegm. Spleen tonics like *dangshen* (党参) are added in the prescription to strengthen spleen *qi* and *chenpi* (陈皮) to improve its flow, consequently strengthening the lung and preventing the production of phlegm. This form of therapy is called tonifying the spleen to promote lung function.

Another example is the treatment of liver *yin* deficiency syndrome with symptoms such dry eyes, vexatiousness, and signs of internal heat. One method of therapy is to nourish the kidney (mother) to promote the liver (child) function, a technique known as 'water nourishing wood' (滋水涵木). Hence, when physicians write prescriptions for this condition, herbs to nourish the kidney *yin* in addition to those that nourish the liver *yin* are used to fortify the liver function.

5

Why We Fall Ill

Diagnosis and principles of therapy

In this chapter we explore the central theme of medicine: what causes illness, how is it diagnosed, and how it is treated.

Why does one fall ill? This may seem a simple question, but the answer is in reality extremely complex. Biomedicine has a branch of study known as etiology which deals with causes of disease, tracing it to microbiological agents like viruses and bacteria and cellular disorders. This kind of approach is considered 'reductionist' because it reduces the explanation of illness to the minutest microscopic factors. Chinese medicine in ancient times did not know of the existence of microbiological agents or understand the functioning of cells. It sought explanation of illness in environmental factors, both internal environmental factors within the body as well as external forces of nature.

Which approach is more correct? Both kinds of explanation are relevant, but TCM chooses to focus on environmental factors. Earlier in Chapter 2, we cited the example of catching the common cold after being exposed to wind and cold weather. The biomedical explanation is that the cold is caused by the common cold virus, whereas TCM focuses on cold and wind pathogens that invade the body and break down its defences. Both explanations are correct, and neither tells the complete story. TCM's focus on environmental factors in practice is useful because it indicates to us that protecting against wind and cold weather and keeping the body's *zhengqi* (正气) strong is the best way to avoid catching colds. The biomedical explanation is technically correct but gives little clue as to how we can prevent colds since the rhinovirus is everywhere in the air.

Let's now examine in more detail the TCM view of various external and internal environmental factors that cause disease.

5.1 Causes of Illness (I): Climatic Factors as Pathogens

Chinese medicine regards the fundamental causes of illness as external climatic factors and internal factors like emotions and poor living habits. In doing so, it takes a more holistic approach to the understanding of causation, focussing not on viruses, bacteria and malfunctioning cells, of which the ancients knew nothing, but on these external and internal environmental factors.

External climatic factors as causes of illness

Climatic factors include six pathogens (*liuyin* 六淫): wind, cold, summer heat, fire, dryness and dampness. These pathogenic factors are closely related to the weather and seasons. Under natural conditions when the body is in harmonious relationship with the nature, these climatic factors do not attack and invade the body to cause illnesses. Only when there is a disruption in harmony with nature, such as being inadequately clothed for the cold weather and the body at the same time is weak and unable to adapt to the seasons or sudden changes in weather, do these climatic factors invade the body and cause illness.

Each climatic factor is prevalent during a certain season. For example, spring tends to be more windy, summer has heat and fire, late summer is damp, autumn is dry and winter is cold. Each climatic factor has its set of characteristics capable of causing illnesses.

Wind tends to float, move and change. Illnesses caused by the wind pathogenic factor are characterised by sudden onset, fast progression and mobility. Mobility has the main symptoms of tremors, dizziness, convulsions or spasms. Often, the site of attack of wind pathogens is at the upper respiratory tract; hence, a common cause for common colds in TCM is wind. For this reason the common cold is also called *shang feng* (伤风), which translates as 'damage by the wind'.

Summer heat tends to dry up the fluids in the body. Hence, typical symptoms of illnesses caused by summer-heat pathogens include thirst, a flushed complexion, sweating, dry stools, high fever, and a fast pulse. Fire has similar characteristics to those of summer heat, the main difference being that the damage by fire is wider and deeper in the body. Fire can lead to wind created internally (endogenous wind) and heat in the blood, and when combined with toxins can result in swelling, ulceration and abscesses.

Dampness has the characteristic of being heavy, sticky and having a tendency to move downward and attack the spleen. Due to its sticky nature, dampness causes stagnation in *qi* and the body consequently develops symptoms such as bloatedness and chest oppression. Other symptoms associated with dampness are sticky loose stools, lethargy, heavy limbs, and a poor appetite. The site of attack is often the abdominal area and the lower trunk of the body.

Dryness tends to attack the lung and dry up body fluids, which explains why most people tend to get dry coughs accompanied with less sputum in the autumn season. Other symptoms associated with dryness are a dry throat, mouth and nose, hard stools and low urine output.

Cold tends to contract, coagulate and destroy *yangqi*. Illnesses caused by cold pathogens usually have symptoms such as pain, aversion to cold and poor *qi* and blood flow.

Falling Ill

Why do some people fall ill while others do not when they are exposed to the same harmful environmental factors? The occurrence of an illness is strongly dependent on our body's state of health, captured by the concept of *zhengqi*, also known as healthy *qi*. When our body is invaded by one of these pathogens, and if the body has strong *zhengqi* we are able to resist and fight off the pathogens. During the battle with the pathogens, our body may warm up and develop symptoms such as fever, a reddish complexion, sweating and phlegm. This condition in which the body generates heat while fighting the invading pathogen is an example of an 'excess' condition, and in TCM it is called an excess syndrome (*shizheng* 实证).

On the other hand, if our *zhengqi* is poor and pathogens attack us, our bodies may succumb to the pathogens and become weaker as the pathogen takes hold. In this weakened condition, we are said to have a 'deficiency condition' or *xuzheng* (虚证). The typical symptoms that are seen in a deficiency condition are lethargy, breathlessness, poor appetite, and a pale complexion.

In sum, the deficiency condition following a pathogenic attack is the result of weakness due to low *zhengqi* yielding to the invading pathogen, whereas an excess condition indicates that the body has an adequate *zhengqi* and is putting up a fight against the pathogen and may well overcome it.

There is a common condition called sub-clinical illness or *yajiankang* (亚健康) (sometimes awkwardly translated as 'sub-health'), in which there is an internal imbalance or poor flows of *qi*, blood or body fluids but there are no obvious clinical symptoms. The person does not feel fully well and experiences various discomforts such as a headache, poor appetite, lassitude, poor sleep. From the biomedical point of view, there are no clinical symptoms of any disease that can be detected through diagnostic tests ordered by the Western doctor and the person is not considered clinically unwell.

However, to the TCM physician he is out of balance and/or experiences impeded flows in the body, and is deemed to have a mild illness and should be treated before the illness develops into something more serious. The World Health Organisation has estimated that up to 80% of people are in the category of sub-clinical illness. One of the relative strengths of TCM is its ability to diagnose sub-clinical illness and prescribe treatments for it. We shall deal with this subject in more depth in a later chapter of the book when we study life cultivation or *yangsheng* (养生).

5.2 Causes of Illness (II): Emotional and Other Internal Factors

In TCM, the emotional factor is very important and many illnesses are in a sense self-inflicted because they result from poor management of our emotions. Unlike the climatic pathogens which are exogenous (external) factors, seven emotions are considered as the endogenous (internal) factors which can cause damage directly to the internal organs. Poor management of a particular emotion is deemed to affect the functions of a particular organ. Too much excitement or overindulgence in joy or sexual pleasure can adversely affect the heart; anger damages the liver; excessive contemplation (thinking excessively and continuously) damages the spleen; grief damages the lung; fear damages the kidney; anxiety damages the lung and liver.

Many of the above emotions are captured in the popular and somewhat loose usage of the word "stress". Depending on the context in which stress is used, it could refer to any one of the above emotions, or a combination of them, although most commonly stress of the kind that is long-term and unremitting tends to be linked to contemplation and anxiety. Contemplation damages the spleen, whilst anxiety and anger hurt the liver which in turn passes it to the spleen and stomach. Hence in high-stress societies like those in Hong Kong, Singapore, Tokyo and New York, disorders of the spleen are especially common as excessive contemplation and anxiety damages the spleen, causing problems of indigestion, irritable bowel syndrome and chronic fatigue.

Working too much or being over-idle are both causes of illness and classified under emotional factors in TCM. Working excessively, too much physical exercise, or over-indulgence in sexual activity strains the body and affects internal flows and balance. For example, overindulgence in sexual activities can harm our kidneys and result in low kidney *qi*, which may affect the urinary function as well as the reproductive system in the long run. Too much idleness such as sitting on the couch and watch television all day will result in poor *qi* and blood flows.

Other Factors

Other causes of illnesses recognised by TCM are improper diet, toxic chemicals and harmful organisms (insects, poisonous animals etc), phlegm and blood stasis. Improper dietary habits can result in dampness and heat in our body and cause stagnation of *qi* of the spleen with the common symptoms of abdominal bloatedness, loose stools, and poor appetite.

We shall talk more about phlegm and blood stasis in the next chapter. Improper diet such as eating too much deep fried and oily food and foods that are strongly flavoured, cold food and drinks, as well as plain gluttony can easily harm our spleen and stomach and result in digestive problems. Toxic chemicals and harmful organisms can cause toxins and heat in our bodies.

5.3 The TCM Syndrome

Earlier in Chapter 2 we touched on the concept of the TCM syndrome (*zheng* 证) as central to TCM thinking about the nature of illness. The TCM syndrome, you will recall, is a group of symptoms forming a pattern that defines the condition of the patient. It should not be confused with the syndrome used in Western medicine, despite superficial similarities.

Chinese medicine recognises syndromes as the basic core of an illness, and the concept of diagnosing and treating syndromes is the essence of TCM. It can be said that TCM focuses on syndromes, whereas Western medicine is more oriented towards diseases. TCM syndromes comprise basic syndromes as well as complex syndromes in which several syndromes are present together.

Basic syndromes are heat, cold, dampness, dryness, deficiency and excess (of *qi*, blood, *yin* or *yang*). Two examples help to illustrate this point.

1. 'Dampness' syndrome is accompanied by a feeling of heaviness in the head, chest oppression, loss of appetite, lassitude, loose stool, sticky fur on the tongue, and a 'soft moderate' pulse (脉濡缓).

2. 'Heat' syndrome is identified by symptoms like aversion to heat, flushed complexion or cheeks, thirst with preference for cold drinks, restlessness/insomnia, yellowish sputum, brownish urine, dry stool, and a reddish tongue. The cause of this syndrome may be an excess of *yang* or deficiency of *yin*.

A complex syndrome can combine several basic syndromes and also be specific to a location. For example, a patient may have the dampness syndrome at the same time the heat syndrome. He is then regarded as having the heat-dampness syndrome, which requires therapy to remove dampness and dispel heat. Just by removing the dampness or heat alone, will not resolve the syndrome. A further complexity would be the heat dampness being specifically located in particular organs, for example heat syndrome of the stomach and spleen. This then requires treatment with herbs that are effective for removing heat and dampness in the spleen and stomach, particularly those herbs with meridian tropism related to the spleen and stomach.

Other examples of complex syndromes are *yin* deficiency of the kidney and *qi* stagnation of the liver with internal heat.

During the progression of an illness, the syndromes are in a dynamic state and will change over time. This explains why it is often not advisable to take the same prescription for a long period of time without consulting the physician as to whether the underlying syndrome of the illness has changed. In this regard, we would like to suggest caution when you go on 'medical visits' organised by guides during your tour of foreign cities where TCM physicians abound. The physician, usually an experienced one who has mastered the art of persuasion, quickly diagnoses your syndromes, tells you that you may be gravely ill and gives a prescription for 6 months or more since you are not visiting him again for a long time. You take home these costly prescriptions and may find that even if they help you initially, after some time your syndromes and conditions would have changed and the huge bag of herbs you brought home may no longer help you.

Phlegm (痰)

Phlegm is considered to be one of the internal factors for the causation of illnesses and is a special type of syndrome. Phlegm usually results from dampness which left untreated progresses to the production of a less viscous fluid called 'rheum' (*yin* 饮), and finally to viscous phlegm. Sticky phlegm is seen as thick mucus that accompanies cough and sneezing. This kind of phlegm is said to have form and substance, as one can see and feel it. In TCM theory, there is another kind of phlegm that is without form. It is the more insidious phlegm that can be challenging to diagnose and treat. It is invisible and persistent and tends to hinder the normal flow of blood and *qi*. It can also cause other symptoms like confusion of mind, chest oppression, numbness in limbs, edema, epilepsy and conditions associated with strokes. In fact, TCM tends to put the blame on such phlegm for causing a variety of illnesses or diseases with no obvious common causes.

Blood Stasis (血瘀)

This results from stagnation in blood and disturbance in circulation, with the production of a pathological substance called blood stasis (*yuxue* 瘀血) that hinders physiological processes. These substances can also be produced by *qi* stagnation (气滞), *qi* deficiency (气虚), blood coldness (血寒), blood heat (血热), trauma or haemorrhage. The blood stasis syndrome is usually manifested as stabbing pain, dark (purple)-coloured tongue, and a thin, taut pulse, and it is one of the more common underlying causes of coronary heart disease.

We shall come across blood stasis often when we study chronic illnesses. Blood stasis is common among patients who have suffered long illness, or who have received severe treatments like chemotherapy and radiation therapy. It tends also to occur more frequently among the elderly.

5.4 TCM Diagnosis

TCM diagnosis differs from western medical diagnosis in relying purely on human observation (visual, tactile, smell, sounds) and the patient's detailed description of his own condition. Through these observations, the physician is able to make inferences regarding the particular syndrome(s) of the patient. Once the syndrome is identified, the physician applies therapeutic principles to formulate a prescription to address the syndrome. This classic process in TCM is known as *bianzhenglunzhi* (辩证论治), which means "identifying the syndrome and treat according to the syndrome." It is the core of Chinese diagnosis and therapy, addressing the illness at its root, and distinguishes it from Western medicine that treats the disease, or sometimes only provides symptomatic relief.

5.4.1 *The four examinations (四诊)*

TCM diagnosis comprises four procedures: inspection (望), smells and sounds (闻), questions (问) and pulsation (切).

Inspection

To inspect means to examine the physical appearance of the patient. This includes looking at the whole body, local regions and the tongue. When we are looking at the whole body, we are trying to obtain general information on the patient by examining his skin complexion, behaviour, posture and most importantly, his eyes which evince the spirit (*shen* 神) of the person, whether they indicate he has good reserves of energy even though he is not feeling well or weak and tired. The body regions for examination refer to a specific part of the body such as the head, hair, five sense organs and neck. It may be necessary even to examine his stool if that is available.

Inspecting the tongue is one of the more important diagnostic tools in Chinese medicine. The colour, shape and flexibility of the tongue reflect the conditions of the viscera (vital organs), *qi* and blood. The fur of the tongue, that is the layer of coating on the tongue which cannot be removed by rinsing the mouth or scraping the tongue, contains information regarding the nature of the pathogenic factors and its interaction with healthy *qi* of the patient. For examples, a red-coloured tongue indicates that there is heat in the body; a pale tongue reflects a deficiency in *qi*, blood or *yang*; and a red tongue with greasy yellow fur points to heat-dampness syndrome in the body.

The tongue of a healthy person should be light reddish in colour with thin white fur. Deviations in the appearance of the tongue and fur from normal are rich in information helping the physician to determine the underlying syndrome(s) of the patient.

Smells and Sounds

These refer to olfaction and listening. The examining physician detects the breath, sputum and mucus, body odour or even the sweat of the patient, and listens to his voice and speech, looking out also for signs of cough, unusual breathing, hiccups and belching. For example, a patient who is coughing very loudly with foul sour-like smell from his sputum usually has heat-phlegm syndrome. On the other hand, when a patient coughs very gently, is soft-spoken and shows breathlessness, it is likely he has a deficiency syndrome.

Questioning

Questioning or interrogation is a crucial basic part of the TCM diagnosis. To ascertain the occurrence, development and treatment of the illness/disease, the physician would inquire into the patient's medical and family history, chief complaint, history of the present illness and current presenting symptoms such as diet, sleep, urination and bowel habits. This is the part of the four examinations from which the physician mines a wealth of information about the patient's condition that will help him greatly to do the diagnosis. Questions to patients in diagnosis are also used by Western doctors although they tend to rely a great on the results of the patient's blood and other diagnostic tests and imaging procedures to aid his diagnosis.

Palpation

Lastly and most often observed by Chinese physicians in movies, pulsation is conducted involving both pulse-taking and palpation. Taking the pulse by placing three fingers over the pulse of the patient helps to reveal more information regarding the inner conditions of the body. When we are taking the pulse, we do not only feel the rate but also the texture and depth. There are altogether 28 pathological pulses in TCM and each pulse has its own specific feel and characteristics relating to one or more types of syndromes. Some of the common pulses encountered in clinical are shown in Table 5.1.

For a complete and accurate TCM diagnosis of the patient, it is necessary for the physician to perform all four examinations

Table 5.1 Varieties of pulse

Pulse	Description	Clinical significance
Floating 浮	Can be felt under light pressure, becomes slightly weak with more pressure	1. External syndrome 2. Internal syndrome due to severe deficiency of blood /essence
Sunken 沉	Can only be felt under heavier pressure	Internal syndrome
Slippery 滑	Smooth like rolling of beads on an abacus	1. Phlegm syndrome 2. Retention of food 3. Sthenic heat syndrome (normal pulse in pregnancy)
Thin or thready 细	Can be felt under light pressure. Weak and thin as a thread	1. Qi and blood deficiency 2. Dampness syndrome
Taut 弦	Feels like the string of a violin	1 Liver and gall bladder disorders 2. Pain 3. Retention of phlegm and fluid

diligently and thoroughly. This information collected will help the physician to differentiate the syndromes so that he can effectively formulate the right therapy to treat the underlying syndromes.

However, the strength of TCM diagnosis is that it is patient-centric, the treatment regime being tailored to the patient rather than the disease itself. Two persons may come in with a cold but based on their presenting symptoms, one may have a heat syndrome whereas the other a cold syndrome. As such, there will be a difference in the treatment. The therapy for the heat syndrome would be to dispel heat whereas that for the cold syndrome it would be to warm the body with suitable medical interventions. This exemplifies the principle that TCM usually treats the syndromes and not the disease directly.

5.4.2 *Syndrome differentiation*

After gathering all the information from the four examinations, the physician then analyses the presenting symptoms, and applying TCM concepts, identifies the pattern. This is also known as "differentiating the syndrome" and indicates to the physician the nature and the underlying cause of the illness. There are several systems of classification of syndromes in TCM. We shall describe here only two main ones used in clinical practice.

The Eight Principles 八纲辩证

A common system of syndrome differentiation in Chinese medicine is the "eight principles" (*bagangbianzheng* 八纲辩证), comprising four pairs of opposite syndromes. These are *yin-yang* 阴阳, external and internal 表里, cold and heat 寒热 and asthenia and sthenia (deficiency and excess) 虚实.

The external and internal principles are used to differentiate the location and stages of the illness, whether it is at the surface/skin level of the body (external) or the imbalances are progressively deeper down to the levels of *qi*, blood and the vital organs (internal). In most cases, external syndromes are at an early stage and are easier to treat to achieve a faster recovery rate whereas internal syndromes tend to take a longer time as they involve treating the impairment of *qi*, body fluids, blood and vital organs, which are necessary for the maintenance of body activities.

The cold and heat principles are used to differentiate the nature of the illness, which actually reflect the level of *yin* and *yang* in the body. As we observed in earlier discussions of TCM syndromes, a heat syndrome is due to an excess of *yang* or deficiency of *yin*. Some symptoms associated with heat syndrome are aversion to heat, flushed complexion or cheeks, thirst with preference for cold drinks, and a red-coloured tongue. On the other hand, a cold syndrome is due to an excess of *yin* or deficiency of *yang*, and some symptoms associated with it are aversion to cold, preference for warmth, cold limbs, a pale complexion, thin clear phlegm, and a light-coloured tongue.

The deficiency and excess principles are used to reflect the state of the healthy *qi* (*zhengqi*) and pathogenic factors. Asthenia, also known as the deficiency syndrome, reflects a weakness in the *zhengqi* when the body is unable to fight off the pathogens. To address this syndrome, the body will need replenishment via the use of tonics. Sthenia, the excess syndrome, is due to an exuberance of pathogenic factors with adequate level of healthy *qi*, when the body is trying to fight off the pathogens. The mode of therapy is to dissipate the pathogens.

You would have noted in the above descriptions that *yin* and *yang* are not only syndromes, but also have an overarching or "umbrella" role as characteristics associated with cold versus heat, internal versus external and deficiency versus excess. This is one of the subtleties of the *yin-yang* concept. It is sometimes used to characterise states of the body like heat and cold, but at other times as syndromes in their own right.

Differentiation by Qi, Blood and Body Fluids

Syndromes can also be differentiated according to whether they are disorders of *qi*, blood or body fluids. Examples of disorders of *qi* are *qi* stagnation and *qi* deficiency syndromes. For blood disorders, there are blood stasis, blood deficiency, and blood-heat syndromes. Body fluids disorders include fluid deficiency and the phlegm syndrome.

Another useful system of classification is by the source of the syndrome, for example dampness, dryness and wind.

In a typical diagnosis, the physician may identify syndromes from the different classifications and apply them to a particular patient. For example, a patient may be differentiated with heat dampness with deficiency of *qi*.

5.5 Therapeutic Principles

After a syndrome is differentiated, we can apply the appropriate therapy to treat the syndromes. The principle involved is to treat a given condition with an opposing and balancing effect. For example:

- Tonify if there is deficiency
- Purge if there is excess
- Cool if there is heat
- Warm if there is cold
- Dry if there is dampness
- Moisten if there is dryness
- Regulate or promote the flow if there is stagnation of *qi*
- Promote blood flow if there is stagnation (stasis) of blood
- Expel if there is wind
- Resolve if there is phlegm

The mode of therapy chosen by the physician can be in the form of herbs, acupuncture, moxibusion or *tuina*, or a combination of either one of these modalities.

We conclude this chapter with an intriguing observation often made of TCM. Sometimes a patient who sees two different physicians may be diagnosed with the same syndromes yet they are treated with different medications. This may happen because there is a certain amount of judgment and experience involved in the choice of therapy. For example, one physician may place more emphasis on making the patient more comfortable earlier by addressing the syndrome that troubles the patient the most, which could be heat. Another physician may prescribe a formulation that is strong in removing dampness as the heat is relatively mild but the dampness is felt to be more serious in the long run in damaging the patient's health.

This phenomenon is not unique to Chinese medicine. Western doctors also often differ in the medications chosen to treat a particular patient's complaints, although for slightly different reasons. With the proliferation of specialisations in Western medicine, each specialist prescribes medications to treat the ailment within his specialty but may add some for other conditions in the patient. When the patient sees another specialist, there is a possibility of that specialist prescribing a different medication for the condition that is used frequently within his specialisation.

Healing the sick is wonderful. But can we go further and find ways to avoid illness and live a long healthy life, perhaps even achieve immortality? That is the subject of the next chapter — seeking the elixir of life.

Chapter

6

Hope Springs Eternal

Ancient wisdom on the elixir of life

The pursuit of the elixir of life has a long history in China. It was an obsession for the great emperor *Qin Shi Huang* (秦始皇) who subdued all warring states in the land and for the first time in history united all of ancient China under one sovereign, so establishing the Qin dynasty (221–207 BC). He was held in awe as much for his military genius as for his unspeakable cruelty, burying alive hundreds of elite Confucian scholars and burning all their books because some of them objected to his lapses in humanity. Everything he fancied in China was for his taking. The only thing that eluded the Qin Emperor and never submitted to him was his mortality.

One after another of his best imperial physicians was executed for failing to produce an elixir of life, the *xiandan* (仙丹) that would enable him to cheat death. Finally, the wiliest of his physicians made a potion with a strong tonic that made him feel invigorated, fooling him that he was on the way to join the ranks of the mythical Taoist immortals, but laced it with enough mercury to kill him slowly. His only remaining claim to immortality is the enormous underground cavern that houses his hidden tomb, guarded by thousands of terracotta soldiers who surely give him comfort that he continues to terrorize the world with bodyguards of fearsome aspect.

The Qin emperor's untimely death just before he turned fifty left behind a power vacuum that swiftly brought an end to the Qin dynasty, which was succeeded by the glorious Han dynasty when the great medical classic *Huangdi Neijing* emerged. The legendary physicians who compiled the *Neijing* declared that man has a natural life span of 100 years, with a few fortunate ones exceeding it by a good margin, but most not even achieving it because most men in the Han era had abandoned the ways of 'the ancients' who preceded them and had mastered the art of living in harmony with nature.

The *Neijing* banished hopes of cheating death but scientists today have revived them as they search for the biological reasons that human beings age and discover drugs that slow down ageing and perhaps one day halt it altogether. They study animals like the crocodile that do not seem to age, capable of living apparently indefinitely for hundreds of years until they get killed by humans, die of disease, or perish from starvation. The new age of a *Back to Methuselah* has began, with the rise of the new science of anti-ageing and the popularity of drugs like Resveratrol, Metformin and Rapamycin that 21st century would-be immortals think will slow down the ageing process by manipulating human genes or intervening in the physiological processes that age body cells.[8] In this mad rush to add those extra years of life on earth, most forget the injunctions of the ancient *Neijing*, that lifespan was always intended to be 100 years — far above what the average person in the developed world can attain — and the best way to achieve it was to stop abusing our bodies and embrace the kind of life our bodies were designed by nature to live.

6.1 The *Neijing* on Living a Long Life

When the *Neijing* opined that man's natural life span was about 100 years, they were not far off the mark by the reckoning of modern physiologists that lifespan is indeed limited by the human cell's ability to regenerate, which declines steadily and comes to a halt after about 100 years. Most men fall short of their natural lifespan because their living habits, physical environments and emotional stress age them prematurely or they die earlier because of preventable conditions like cardiovascular disease and cancer.

As far back as two thousand years ago the *Neijing* lamented that the modern man of those times, compared to the ancients hundreds or thousands of years before, had departed from the rules of healthy living. In a celebrated passage on the art of cultivating the good life, the *Neijing* declares:

> The ancients knew the *tao* and understood the principles of yin and yang, and practised exercises of body and mind. They observed

---

[8] See, for example, "Cheating Death", London: *The Economist*, 13 August 2016, pp. 9 and 16–18.

moderation and appropriateness of diet, kept regularity in living habits, avoided over-exertion, and achieved harmony of body and spirit.[9]

The wisdom of the *Neijing* is encapsulated in these simple lines containing just 30 Chinese characters. They would appear easy or simple to follow, but in practice require so much self-discipline and understanding of medical principles that few can fully meet its injunctions.

The '*tao*' in the text means the proper of approach to conducting one's life, and is not a direct reference to Taoism, although the allusion to it is likely as Taoists were known to have mastered the art of longevity.

The principle of *yin* and *yang* and the achievement of harmony through balance and flows are cardinal principles of cultivating health, as we observed in Chapter 2 of the book.

The exercises of body and mind known as *shushu* are an ancient art involving subtle movements with meditative mind involvement, somewhat similar to their modern counterparts found in various form of *qigong* exercises.

"Moderation and appropriateness of diet" implies not over-eating (80 percent full is healthier than a full stomach); using moderate quantities of various kinds of food and eating the right foods appropriate to one's constitution and season of the year. The right diet would include herbs to balance the body, tonic herbs to fortify the *zhengqi* of the body, and herbal supplements that promote the flow of qi, blood and body fluids.

Regularity in living habits included rising in the morning and retiring to bed at fixed times according to the seasons, eating regular meals at about the same time, and working hours that follow patterns dictated by the climate and time of the year. Such regularity makes for optimal functioning of the body,

---

[9]The Chinese text puts it succinctly: "上古之人, 其知道者; 法于阴阳, 和与术数. 饮食有节, 起居有常. 不妄作劳, 故能形与神俱."

actively working or exercising when *yangqi* is abundant, as in early morning and early afternoon, preparing to rest in the early evening when the *yin* cycle of the day takes over and reaches a peak at midnight.

The importance of regularity has been noted by Western observers. The greatest of German philosophers Immanuel Kant (1724–1804) was known to been a creature of habit, adhering religiously to schedules for such mundane activities as rising from bed and taking his morning walk at such precise times of the day that his neighbours would set their clocks according to the time the learned Immanuel walked past their windows. We do not know whether Kant followed the *Neijing* on diet, over-exertion and exercise, but regularity alone seemed to have helped him immensely to attain the age of 80, unusual for his generation.

Modern physiologists know that sleeping early allows the body to repair itself efficiently and facilitates the function of the liver in this process. Poor observance of regularity by top executives, missing lunches and dining late as business meetings require, would appear to be correlated with their higher incidence of pancreatic cancer as the pancreas is known to be more sensitive to irregular cycles upsetting its sugar regulating functions.[10]

Finally, maintaining healthy emotions so that the body and spirit are working smoothly together in harmony is the *Neijing* passage's most important instruction. So crucial is this injunction to attaining health that dozens of eminent scholar-physicians over centuries have written extensively on the practical means of working through its implications. The Chinese leisure pursuits of the cultured man, comprising calligraphy, painting,

---

[10] Steve Jobs of Apple Inc. arguably may have been a victim of this.

playing the musical instrument *qin*, and chess are but means of attaining such serenity.

In subsequent chapters of this book, as we gain more knowledge of TCM, we shall learn how to apply the principles of health preservation in the *Neijing* through various *yangsheng* practices and the enjoyment of nourishing medicated foods, teas and soups for promoting health and longevity. We shall also discuss the ideas of renowned practitioners of *yangsheng* who drew on the wisdom of the *Neijing* and extended it by adapting to the physical environment, culture and society.

6.2 Avoiding Illness

Another famous passage from the *Neijing* concerns the avoidance of illness:

> If you avoid climatic stresses, live a placid life with plain needs, maintain defensive forces in the body, and keep yourself in good spirits, how then could you possibly fall ill? [11]

As we saw in the last chapter, the causes of illness in Chinese holistic thinking lie principally in natural climatic forces and excessive emotions. This is succinctly captured in *Neijing*'s advice on avoiding illness.

The passage also puts the responsibility of disease prevention squarely on each person's own lifestyle and attitude to life, and in startlingly simple terms: lead a placid life and keep good spirits.

A placid life with plain needs is conducive to avoiding the unremitting corroding effects of excessive contemplation and anxiety on the spleen and liver. Digestive problems like acid

---

[11] "虚邪贼风,避之有时,恬淡虚无,真气从之,精神内守,病安从来。"

reflux, bloated stomachs, loss of appetite, stomach ulcers and the irritable bowel syndrome are rampant in high achievement-oriented societies. Modern treatment with antacids, proton pump inhibitors and various medications to reduce inflammation and stomach secretions only help control the symptoms but do not offer relief at the more basic level of the underlying causes. To alleviate these conditions, TCM would attack these problems at the level of their syndromes like impeded flows of liver *qi* and deficiency of spleen *qi* exacerbated by dampness.

While these remedies may provide more satisfactory relief at the root level, it does not solve the problem permanently unless an even more fundamental problem is addressed, that of the stresses of modern living. To understand this point, we need only witness the way of life of people who live in Buettner's 'Blue Zones' like Okinawa, Japan and Ikaria, Greece. In these special regions of the world, there is a high proportion of centenarians living active healthy lives right up to the final months of their lives. A consistent pattern can be seen: these people lead simple and placid lives, at peace with a plain existence in socially supportive communities where family and friends gather daily to share their joys and worries and feel a warm sense of belonging to a close-knit group.[12]

---

[12] Buetter, D (2008) *The Blue Zones.* Washington: National Geographic.

7

Nature's Goodness in a Humble Root

The nature and flavour of herbs

The humble root of a plant, or its leaves, bark, flowers and seeds all have potential medicinal value. Many of these plant parts have been carefully studied for their health promotion and therapeutic effects, and recorded in the Chinese pharmacopeia compiled over thousands of years by generations of herbalists and physicians.

The earliest extant manual on herbs was based on the work of Shen Nong containing detailed descriptions of 365 herbs that he personally tested for toxicity and side effects. The most comprehensive record of Chinese herbs to date, was first published in 1578 during the Ming dynasty, and has since then served as a reference text by Chinese physicians and pharmacists. The *Compendium of Materia Medica (Bencao Gangmu* 本草纲目*)* covered 1892 items, inclusive of medicines of animal and mineral origins. This encyclopaedic scholarly work based on patient and meticulous studies and experimentation is lasting testimony to the empirical scientific tradition in Chinese medicine. TCM relies on clinical evidence provided by detailed observation, record and analysis, and although its methods may differ from those of modern biomedicine, it is no less rooted in empirical science.

In modern times, most Chinese herbs have been analysed in the laboratory and in clinical trials for therapeutic properties, toxicity and side effects and the accumulation of these studies and the experience of earlier generations of physicians have been carefully documented in modern texts on Chinese medicinal herbs. Much work remains to be done as the variety of herbs is very large and their complexity is of a much higher order than modern pharmaceuticals. Just a single herb typically contains dozens and sometimes over a hundred different ingredients and molecules in contrast to a Western drug that comprises a single chemical known as its active ingredient.

Whenever we think about Chinese medicine herbs, we tend to relate them to a bitter concoction that takes about an hour or so to boil. Although most of the herbs are prepared this way for consumption to bring about the required therapeutic effects, many medicinal herbs such as Chinese yam, *dangshen* (党参), *yuzhu* (玉竹), gingko, and lily bulb are regularly used as food ingredients in daily family meals. Such herbs are favoured for cooking as they are more pleasant to taste and can serve both as medicine as well as sources of nutrition. There is indeed no strict distinction between herbs and foods as medicine. In Chapter 11 of the book, we shall delve into the exciting and mouth-watering world of combining herbs into daily cooking in diets for a healthy lifestyle.

7.1 Sources and Classification of Herbs

Plant sources of herbs include roots, grasses, leaves, barks, stems, flowers, seeds and fruits. For example, ginseng and Chinese angelica (*danggui* 当归) are roots; chrysanthemum and honeysuckle are flowers; peppermint is a leaf; wolfberries are fruits and *duzhong* (杜仲) is from the bark of a tree.

Medicines can also be derived from minerals and animals. Mineral sources include oyster shells, magnetite and haematite. Even creatures like scorpions, centipedes and silkworms are usable as medicine; parts of animals such as the tortoise shell and a gelatine made from donkey skin (*ejiao* 阿胶) are surprisingly valuable as tonics for nourishing the *yin* and commonly used in concoctions for improving the complexion.

For ease of reference, all medicinal ingredients used in TCM will be termed 'herbs' in this book. In a more formal academic context, the correct term Chinese *materia medica* (中药) should be used.

The study of Chinese herbs is a vast and complex enterprise, so rich is the source of materials with medicinal qualities. Each herb of plant or animal origin is part of a living thing and not a mere chemical.

Even the humble orange has many different components each with different properties and healing capabilities. In everyday living we tend to look at the orange as a source of Vitamin C, some fibre and mineral salts. However in Chinese medicine, even the dried skin of a special variety of orange or tangerine known as *juzi* (橘子) (*citrus reticulate Blanco*) has amazing healing properties. When dried and kept for a period of time in storage, the orange skin is known as *chenpi* (陈皮), used largely to aid the movement of *qi* (regulating *qi* in TCM terminology). It is therefore helpful for resolving phlegm caused by dampness which tends to impede the flow of *qi*. But studies have shown that *chenpi* may also have vasodilating properties and improving blood flow, and also in the reduction of triglycerides in the blood. Hence a mere tangerine can have many medicinal uses when applied to different conditions.

Likewise the herb *huangqi* (黄芪) or *astragalus,* among the most widely used of Chinese herbs, is principally a *qi* tonic, but it has many other useful properties such as promoting diuresis and strengthening the body's defence system. Some studies have shown it may help increase white blood cell and platelet count and it is to be found in prescriptions for patients after chemotherapy or radiotherapy who suffer declines in these blood components. *Astragalus* is also thought to have life-extension properties as it can stimulate the lengthening of the teleomerase in the human cell DNA that is involved in cell regeneration. We shall occasion to mention this again in a later chapter of the book when we discuss Chinese secrets of longevity.

Each Chinese herb being so complex and having many medicinal properties, how does Chinese medicine go about classifying herbs? Scholars and physicians over time have agreed on a system of classification by which the herb's most common use is taken into account. For example, *chenpi* is classified as a herb for regulating *qi* and *huangqi* as a *qi* tonic. Hence herbs are classified by their therapeutic actions; we shall discuss these in the next chapter. Before that, we should also look at classifying herbs according to property (nature) and flavour (taste), as these are also important indicators of how the herbs can be used for medical purposes in practice. Another aspect of herbs is that they have a tendency to be more effective when applied to certain meridians; this phenomenon is known as meridian tropism (*guijing* 归经), and will also be discussed further below.

7.2 Properties of Herbs

The property of a herb refers to its nature, whether it has a warming or cooling effect on the body; the usual classifications are hot, warm, neutral, cool and cold. Excluding the neutral property, these are also known as "the four natures" or *siqi* (四气). The property attributed to herb derives from its effect on pathogenic heat and cold. Therefore, herbs that are warm in nature, such as cinnamon, have a warming effect on the body and are used to treat cold syndromes, whereas herbs with cool property, such as chrysanthemum flower, are used to treat heat syndromes by dispelling heat pathogens. Herbs that are hot have stronger effects than warm herbs and are often used to treat more severe cold syndromes such as kidney *yang* deficiency. Being hotter in nature, if used inappropriately they are more inclined to produce troublesome side effects of internal heat with symptoms such as constipation and a sore throat. Dried ginger is an example of a hot herb.

Conversely, herbs that are cold in nature have stronger cooling actions than herbs that are cool, hence, they are used to treat severe heat syndromes such as exuberance of stomach fire. Inappropriate or excess usage of cold herbs over a prolonged period of time can damage the spleen by impairing spleen *yang* and giving rise to symptoms such as loose stools, aversion to cold and poor appetite. A common herb with cold property is gypsum (*shigao* 石膏).

As the name implies, herbs that are neutral in nature are neither hot nor cold and can be used in both heat and cold syndromes. The therapeutic actions for this group of herbs are generally milder and do not have any contraindications. As they are suitable for most people with different constitutions, they are also very suitable for use as foods. Examples of neutral herbs are the Chinese yam and liquorice roots (甘草 *gancao*).

It should be noted that these classifications are of a general nature and may not always apply rigidly to different individuals with varying constitutions. Some persons who have warm constitutions may react to warm herbs as if they were hot; a herb like the American ginseng root is normally classified as cool, but there are people who find it a little warm or 'heaty'. Hence the physician needs to exercise some discretion in prescribing herbs after taking into account the physical condition of his patient. Nevertheless the classifications are extremely useful guides in practice.

7.3 Flavours

The flavour of a herb, used as a TCM term, is akin to its taste, except that in Chinese medicine certain actions are associated with the flavour classification, hence there is not always an exact correspondence between the flavour and taste of a herb. Each herb can have more than one flavour. The five flavours are pungent (辛), sweet (甘), bitter (苦), sour (酸), and salty (咸) (Table 7.1).

Herbs that are pungent usually have the actions of dispersing and promoting *qi* and blood flow. In Chinese medical terms, to disperse is to dispel the pathogens from the body surface and that is usually done through sweating. Most herbs that are used to treat exogenous (external) syndromes are pungent. Examples of herbs that are pungent are the chrysanthemum flower and mulberry leaves.

Table 7.1   Herbal flavours

Flavours	Functions	Examples
Pungent 辛	• Dispersion 解表	*Bohe* (Peppermint) 薄荷
Sweet 甘	• Nourishes 补 • Replenishes 润 • Harmonizes 和	*Gancao* (Liquorice) 甘草
Sour 酸	Arresting 收敛固涩	*Wuweizi* 五味子
Bitter 苦	• Clearing heat 泻火 • "Sending down" adverse flows of *qi* 降逆	*Xiakucao* 夏枯草
Salty 咸	• Purges 泻下 • Softens 软坚	*Mangxiao* 芒硝

Herbs that are sweet have the actions of nourishing, moistening and harmonising; this is seen in most tonics, which are a group of herbs used to treat syndromes of deficiency in *qi*, blood, *yin* or *yang*. Ginseng, wolfberries and red dates are examples of tonics that are sweet. Liquorice (甘草) is the only tonic that also has a harmonising action. It is used in most formulations with the aim to harmonise or regulate the actions of the other herbs in the prescription.

The actions of herbs classified as bitter are heat clearing and drying, which means that heat-clearing herbs are cool or cold in nature and are used to treat heat syndromes. One of the modes of expelling or purging the heat/fire is through urination or defecation. Some examples of heat-clearing herbs are *xiakucao* (夏枯草) and *dahuang* (大黄).

Herbs that are sour have arresting action which means that they are used to treat excessive loss of body fluids from profuse sweating, diarrhea, frequent urination, and excessive white discharge or seminal fluids. An example is *wuweizi* (五味子).

Lastly, the effect associated with being salty is softening of hard nodules and masses, and promoting defecation. One example is *mangxiao* (芒硝).

Some herbs have a combination of flavours. For example tangerine peel *chenpi* is classified as pungent and bitter, giving it the action of drying as well as promoting *qi* flow to resolve dampness, and hence its use in cough medications to treat the dampness syndrome.

Herbs with a drying action are usually warm.

7.4 Meridian Tropism

Each herb is thought to have one or more preferential routes along the meridians for their actions to affect specific organs; this is termed meridian tropism. For example, wolfberry is associated with liver, kidney and lung meridians hence is used in formulations for eyesight (associated with liver), tinnitus (kidney) and certain coughs (lung).

As stated earlier, most herbs have several therapeutic actions even though they are classified into different categories based on their main action. In Chinese medicine, most herbs have more than one flavour and more than one preferred meridian associated with their therapeutic actions. However, each herb can only have one nature which will determine its application on either heat or cold syndrome. From the biomedical perspective, this is because a herb contains a large variety of components and molecules, and its action cannot be captured by just one classification.

7.5 Toxicity

What does it mean for a herb to be toxic? This is important to understand because this term is sometimes abused and misunderstood.

'Toxic' in Western medicine means having a poisonous effect, i.e. it impairs the body tissues. The term is "usually reserved for substances (like arsenic)…that are harmful in small amounts."[13] In other words, toxic substances like arsenic and mercury if taken in even small or moderate quantity can cause bad reactions, illnesses or death.

However, in Chinese medicine, the word toxic or *du* (毒) has a wider meaning and only one of these meanings corresponds to its use in Western medicine. Examples of its other meanings are as follows.

(a) It has special use for fighting pathogens, e.g. dried ginger against cold pathogens. In this case, this toxicity is directed at the pathogens. Of course when it kills the pathogens it will sometimes have harmful side effects on the body and should be used with caution.

(b) Toxicity could mean an undesirable side effect e.g. *shexiang* (麝香) (musk) for resuscitation and blood circulation (to remove masses) can induce abortion. Used in the right amount, it can provide the desired therapeutic effects, but in excess it would cause harm.

(c) Excessive use is harmful e.g. apricot kernel (*ku xingren* 苦杏仁) has traces of cyanide. In practice, the bitter *xingren* is used within a certain dosage limit.

There is a saying in Chinese that says "use poison to fight poison" (以毒攻毒) and "attack pathogens with poisonous herbs"(毒药攻邪); these meanings are mainly related to (a) above. It means that something you have to take may be directed to a pathogen even though it may have side effects to the body. Generally, Chinese medicine herbs are quite safe to consume if they are collected from the right sources and used in correct

---

[13] *Oxford Medical Dictionary*, 4th edition (2007).

dosages. In fact, the majority of the herbs that are found in Chinese medical halls are processed, which means that the level of toxicity in herbs is greatly reduced to a safe level for consumption after boiling.

7.6 Processing of Herbs

We can hardly find raw herbs in most medical halls nowadays as most of them would have gone through some forms of processing when they are offered for retail. There are many types of processing methods, which would include baking, stir-frying, washing, burning, calcination, simmering, and steaming. The purpose for processing herbs includes

(a) Removing or reducing toxicity e.g. *fuzi* (附子) requires to be boiled separately for at least 1 hour before mixing with other herbs.
(b) Promoting or enhancing the therapeutic effect e.g when safflower (*honghua* 红花) is soaked in wine, it has a stronger effect in its blood promoting action
(c) Modifying nature and actions: *shengdihuang* (生地黄) is cool and is used for clearing heat and cooling the blood but after it has undergone cooking in wine, it becomes *shudihuang* (熟地黄) (cooked *rehemmania*). Its property changes from cool to slightly warm, making it suitable for nourishing blood. Both *shengdihuang* and *shudihuang* are also used in combination with herbs for nourishing *yin*.
(d) Facilitating decocting and ingestion of medicine, preparation and storage by cutting the herbs into smaller pieces and drying them in the sun or baking them. These procedures will help to prolong the storage life of the herbs while maintaining their properties. For example, silkworms (*jiangcan* 僵蚕) are usually stir-fried in salt so as to extend its

shelf-life. Mineral herbs like oyster shells will need to undergo burning, soaking them in vinegar and crushing for easy dispensing and, most importantly, to allow easy extraction of the active ingredients upon brewing with other herbs in the formulation.

(e) Removing impurity and unpleasant tastes.

7.7 Compatibility of Herbs

A TCM formulation usually comprises several herbs and it is important to know how to combine the herbs effectively to increase the efficacy of the therapy, and how they are combined depends on the compatibility of the herbs with one another. In other words, certain herbs can work together to enhance a particular therapeutic action whereas certain herbs cannot and may produce serious side effects if they are used together in the same formulation. Below are some of the rules of herbs compatibility that are practiced in Chinese medicine.

(a) Mutual reinforcement (*xiangxu* 相须): The herbs are compatible with one another and by putting them together; it reinforces the therapeutic action of one another. Herbs which are in this relationship usually have similar properties and actions. For example, safflower (*honghua* 红花) and peach seed (*taoren* 桃仁) are both blood promoting herbs and they are usually used together to reinforce their actions of enhancing blood flow and removing blood stasis. As a result, the effect of promoting blood flow is stronger as compared to just using either one of the herbs alone.

(b) (Mutual) assistance (*xiangshi* 相使): The herbs do not have similar properties and their main therapeutic actions differ. One herb will be the principal herb and is used for its main therapeutic action while the other herb is used as an assisting role to enhance the main therapeutic action of the principal herb. For example, *huangqi* (黄芪) (the principal herb) which is a *qi* tonic is used to replenish spleen *qi* and poria (茯苓) (the assistant herb), which is a diuretic with some mild *qi*-tonifying action, is used to enhance *huangqi's* action for reducing water retention arising from the spleen-*qi* deficiency syndrome.

(c) (Mutual) restraint/detoxification (*xiangwei/xiangsha* 相畏/相杀): One herb reduces or removes the side effects or toxicity of another herb. For example, raw ginger (*shengjiang* 生姜) reduces the toxicity of *banxia* (半夏).

(d) (Mutual) inhibition (*xiange* 相恶): In this relationship, the combination of the herbs will produce an undesirable effect, in which one reduces the effectiveness of the other. For example, the therapeutic action of ginseng (人参) is weakened by radish (*laifuzi* 莱菔子). Therefore, these two herbs are not used together in a prescription.

(e) Incompatibility (*xiangfan* 相反) is a combination of two herbs that will result in toxicity. There are a total of such 18 cases recorded in the Chinese pharmacopeia. One such pair is *wutou* (乌头) and *beimu* (贝母).

7.8 Contraindications

As in Western medicine, there are contraindications when taking Chinese medicine herbs. This means that the herbs should be taken with caution under medical supervision in certain situations as illustrated below:

During pregnancy, toxic herbs and herbs that are used for promoting blood flow and removing blood stasis should be used with caution as the enhanced blood flow may be too strong for the uterus, resulting in risk of miscarriage. Examples of such herbs are *shexiang, honghua, dahuang* and *fuzi*.

People with weak digestive systems are more sensitive to herbs that are of cool or cold in nature as these herbs tend to impair their spleen and stomach functions by damaging *yang*, and causing symptoms such as poor appetite, loose stools, pain or discomfort in the gastric upon taking cold food. Examples of such herbs are *huangqin* (黄芩), *dahuang*, and gypsum.

It is always advisable not to take tonics when one is having the flu or a fever. This is because tonics are mostly warm or hot in nature and taking them during fever will worsen the condition. The saying in Chinese medicine "闭门留寇" means "close the door and trap the intruder," implying that tonics have a similar effect to closing the door and keeping the intruder inside the house. Similarly, taking tonics when having an infectious cold is like providing the invaded pathogens more nourishment to thrive and cause harm to our body.

7.9 Dosage

The dosage of herbs to be taken by patient is often decided by the physician based on the patient's condition, constitution, and history. This explains why it is always safer to consult a physician before taking medications. For example, more heat-clearing herbs should be given to someone who has a warm body constitution or suffering from a heat syndrome as compared to someone who has a cold body constitution or weak digestive system. In the case of the latter, the dosage of heat-clearing herbs to be given should be lower and be prescribed for a shorter period of time.

In general, it is advisable for tonics to be taken before meals; herbs that may upset the stomach should be taken after meals, and calmatives before sleep.

7.10 Preparation of Herbs for Decoctions

Depending on the type of herbs, different herbs may require different methods of preparation. Herbs that are toxic such as *fuzi* will require prior boiling for one to one and a half hours to remove the toxins before cooking it with other herbs; herbs that contain volatile components such as peppermint and *gouteng* (钩藤) should only be boiled in the last five or ten minutes so that the heat will not disperse its volatile components and destroy the ingredients with therapeutic actions. Herbs that are hairy in shape or come in very fine particles will need to be isolated in sachets from the other herbs as remnants floating in the decoction may irritate the throat. Examples are *cheqianzi* (车前子) and *xuanfuhua* (旋覆花).

8

Potions That Heal

Herbs and herbal formulations

We now turn to the practical reason for studying herbs: how to use them to heal illness and to promote health. This is a vast and fascinating area of study, taught in medical universities as an important subject but also as degree and research courses entirely devoted to studying their healing actions.

In this chapter, we first look at how to classify herbs according to their therapeutic actions before discussing how they can be combined into formulations (like cocktails) for wider and more potent or effective use.

8.1 Classification of Herbs by Action

The main classifications are listed below:

1. Diaphoretics (*jiebiao yao* 解表药): removing either warm or cold pathogens at the surface (exterior) level
2. Heat-clearing (*qingre yao* 清热药): clearing internal heat
3. Purgatives (*xiexia yao* 泻下药): lubricating the large intestine or inducing diarrhoea to move bowel and relieve constipation
4. Removing dampness (*qushi yao* 祛湿药): eliminating dampness within the body and promoting diuresis
5. Warming interior (*wenli yao* 温里药): warms interior of body and dispels cold
6. Regulating *qi* (*liqi yao* 理气药): promoting the movement of *qi*
7. Relieving food retention (*xiaoshi yao* 消食药): helping in digestion and relieving food retention
8. Invigorating blood and removing stasis (*huoxue huayu yao* 活血化瘀药): promoting better blood flow and removing stasis
9. Resolving phlegm (*huatan yao* 化痰药): removing phlegm in the body
10. Tranquilisers (*anshen yao* 安神药): calming the mind
11. Calming liver and wind (*pinggan xifen yao* 平肝熄风药): calming the liver and suppressing hyperactive *yang*, or calming liver wind
12. Tonics (restoratives) (*buyi yao* 补益药): tonics for *qi*, blood, *yin* and *yang*
13. Astringents (*shoulian gushe yao* 收敛固摄药): arresting excessive discharge of fluids such as perspiration, diarrhoea and urine

14. Hemostatic herbs (*zhixue yao* 止血药): assist in stopping bleeding, internally and externally, by cooling the blood, warming the channels or by astringent action
15. Eliminating parasites (*qucong yao* 驱虫药)

A list of common herbs with descriptions of their nature, properties and principal applications is provided in Annex 1. We select below a number of classifications that are more commonly used in clinical practice.

8.1.1 *Diaphoretics* (解表药)

Diaphoretics are used to treat exogenous (external) syndromes. Most of them are pungent in flavour which explains why their main therapeutic action is to disperse the exogenous pathogens, mainly through sweating. Their preferences are mostly the lung and bladder meridians. Based on their nature, diaphoretic herbs can be further divided into two categories: herbs with pungent-warm properties and herbs with pungent-cool properties. Diaphoretics which are pungent-warm are used to treat exogenous cold syndromes whereas pungent-cool diaphoretics are used for exogenous heat syndromes.

Examples of diaphoretic with pungent-warm properties are *Ephedra sinica* (*mahuang* 麻黄) and *Cinnamomum cassia* (*guizhi* 桂枝). These herbs are mutually compatible and often used together to treat exogenous cold syndromes by inducing sweating to expel the wind-cold pathogens. They share a mutual reinforcement relationship. Additional actions of *ephedra* include promoting diuresis and dispersing the lung to relieve breathlessness; for cinnamon, it is also sometimes used to warm the collaterals and heart *yang*.

Examples of diaphoretics with pungent-cool properties are chrysanthemum flower (*juhua* 菊花) and mulberry leaves (*sangye* 桑叶). These two herbs also share a mutual reinforcement relationship and are often used together in a formulation called *sangjuyin* 桑菊饮 to treat cough resulted from exogenous wind-heat pathogens. In other words, it is used to treat coughs which are in the initial stage when it is still accompanied by other flu-like symptoms such as a running nose, chills, and headache. Other than using them to treat coughs at the initial stage, we can also use them together to clear internal liver fire as indicated by their bitter flavour. Therefore, they can be used in conditions such as red and sore eyes, poor vision or headache resulted from liver fire. These are some of the few diaphoretics that can expel both exogenous and internal heat.

There are several varieties of chrysanthemum flowers and they share similar actions although one may have a stronger effect in a certain action. For example, yellow chrysanthemum flowers (*huangju* 黄菊) have a stronger effect in dispersing wind-heat pathogens whereas white chrysanthemum flowers (*baijun/hanju* 白菊/杭菊) are often used for clearing liver fire and suppressing hyperactivity of liver *yang*; it is also often the popular choice for making teas due to its sweet fragrance. Another type, known as the wild chrysanthemum flower (*yejuhua* 野菊花), has the additional action of clearing toxins. They come in smaller sizes and are often used to treat carbuncles, acnes, sores, ulcers etc resulted from heat-toxin syndrome. In addition to having the heat-clearing and expelling actions of mulberry leaves, it also has a moistening action which chrysanthemum flowers do not have. Therefore, mulberry leaves are sometimes used in dry coughs to help moisten and nourish the lung *yin*.

8.1.2 *Heat-clearing herbs* (清热药)

Heat-clearing herbs group comprises many herbs and is one of the biggest classifications in the Chinese pharmacopeia. As implied by the name, the main action of the herbs is to clear heat; and the properties for this group are cold/cool and bitter. These herbs should not be taken for too long and an individual with a weak spleen and stomach should take them with caution due to their cold nature.

Within this classification, there are other sub-categories such as heat-clearing and purging fire (清热泻火), heat-clearing and resolving dampness (清热燥湿), heat-clearing and blood cooling (清热凉血), heat-clearing and detoxification (清热解毒) and clearing asthenic heat (清虚热).

Some of the common heat-clearing herbs used in the tropics are honeysuckle flower, *lianqiao* (连翘), *xiakucao* (夏枯草) and *chuanxinlian* (穿心莲). Honeysuckle flower (*jinyinhua* 金银花) is a heat-clearing and detoxification herb, which is often used to treat carbuncles, acnes, and ulcers. It can also expel exogenous wind-heat pathogens and is one of the principal herbs used in the formulation *yinqiaosan* (银翘散), in which the other principal herb is *lianqiao*. This formulation is used to treat initial stage of exogenous wind-heat syndrome which has symptoms such as fever, chills, sore throat, thirst and headache. Tea with honeysuckle flower helps to soothe a mild sore throat and feeling of an imminent common cold. In comparison to the honeysuckle flower, *chuanxinlian* has stronger heat-clearing and detoxification actions. In addition, it has blood cooling action which helps to reduce swelling. Therefore, *chuanxinlian* is often used to treat more severe cases of internal heat syndrome which includes dysentery, abscess, and insect and animal bites.

8.1.3 *Purgatives* (泻下药)

Purgatives are a group of herbs that help to stimulate evacuation of bowels either by inducing laxative effects or moistening large intestines to promote bowel movement. However, it is not advised to use these herbs for prolong period of time as it will result in diarrhea and lead to dehydration. We should stop taking these herbs once bowel movement is normal. Pregnant women, elderly and people with weak digestive systems should either avoid taking these herbs or take it with caution because of their strong actions. *Dahuang* (大黄) has the properties of cold and bitter and it is used to treat constipation associated with the sthenic heat syndrome as the underlying cause. Main symptoms manifested are hard stools, difficulty in emptying the bowels, stomach pain, accompanied by other heat symptoms such as thirst, bad breath and a red tongue. *Dahuang* also helps to promote blood and remove stasis hence this herb should be avoided during pregnancy, menstruation and lactation. Purgatives that help to moisten the large intestines are mostly seeds as they have high oil content which helps to provide lubrication to the movement of bowels along the intestines. One example is *huomaren* (火麻仁), often used to treat constipation due to blood or fluid deficiency syndrome. Its purgative effect is much milder than that of *dahuang*, hence it is suitable to use on pregnant women and elderly.

8.1.4 *Qi-regulating herbs* (理气药)

Qi regulating herbs are mostly warm and pungent in flavour and their main action is to promote *qi* flow. One very common example is dried tangerine peel (*chenpi* 陈皮). It is used to treat spleen and stomach *qi* stagnation which cause abdominal bloatedness. In most cases of spleen *qi* stagnation, the main culprit is dampness as we know that one of its characteristics is sticky and tends to impair the *qi* flow. Therefore, herbs that help to regulate *qi* in the spleen usually have another action of drying dampness which is that of *chenpi*. *Chenpi* also helps to resolve wet phlegm and can be used to treat cough due to cold or wet phlegm syndrome.

Another *qi* regulating herb which is commonly known to many people as a love flower is the rose. Most people may not realise that rose actually helps to regulate the flow of liver *qi* and also promote blood flow to relieve pain. In fact, with better liver *qi* and blood flows, rose can help to enhance one's complexion as more *qi* and blood can reach our skin to nourish them.

8.1.5 *Diuretics and herbs that remove dampness* (利水渗湿药)

Diuretics are a group of herbs that promote urination to remove dampness and excess water from the body, and are often used to treat edema (water retention). One common example is Chinese barley, which is also known as the Job's tears (*yiyiren* 薏苡仁). This should be distinguished from English barley, which is smaller in size and has different properties. Chinese barley may be consumed when one feels 'heaty'. This is because it is cool in nature and has the action of clearing heat and draining dampness by promoting urination. In fact, *yiyiren* tea or dessert is suitable to drink in the tropics due to the humid weather. Raw *yiyiren* is cooler and clears heat better than stir-fried *yiyiren*, which is slightly warmer, and is usually used to treat diarrhea caused by spleen-*qi* deficiency.

Poria, *fuling* (茯苓), on the other hand is neutral in nature, and hence can be used in most syndromes, regardless of heat or cold syndromes. Besides promoting urination to drain dampness and relieve water retention, it has the mild effect on tonifying spleen *qi* and calming the mind.

8.1.6 *Herbs for promoting blood flow* (活血化瘀药)

Herbs for promoting blood flow and removing stasis are mainly attributed to the liver and heart meridians, and they are mostly warm, pungent and bitter. This group of herbs is often used to relieve pain and regulate menstruation, and should be used with caution for pregnant women.

Chuanxiong (川芎) helps to promote both blood and *qi* flow, and is used to treat pain arising from cold syndrome which results in *qi* stagnation and blood stasis. It is also one of the herbs used in the formulation *siwutang* (四物汤) which is used for treating blood deficiency syndrome. Based on past experience and records, *chuanxiong* is regarded as being good at relieving headaches and is quite commonly used in clinical practice.

Another example is *danshen* (丹参) which has a slightly different property from the rest of the blood promoting herbs as it is cool in nature instead of being warm like most herbs in this category. Due to its cool nature, *danshen* has the action of cooling the blood to promote healing of abscess, as well as, soothing irritability and calming the mind, and can be used to treat insomnia arising from blood heat syndrome. *Danshen* is more commonly used to treat menstruation problems such as irregularity, cramps and low menstruation volume because it helps to regulate better blood circulation. Recent clinical studies suggest that *danshen* can dilate coronary arteries, and it is now one of the principal herbs used in *fufang danshendiwan* (复方丹参滴丸) used to treat mild coronary heart disease.

8.1.7 *Hemostatic herbs* (止血药)

Herbs that can stop internal and external bleeding are known as hemostatic herbs.

Pseudoginseng, also commonly known as *sanqi* (三七) or *tianqi* (田七), is the most common example. It helps to stop bleeding by removing blood stasis and promoting blood flow. *Sanqi* is given the name pseudoginseng because it is strictly not a *qi* tonic like ginseng but it mimics its *qi* tonifying action by not damaging the *zhengqi* (healthy *qi*) of the body when promoting blood flow, which most blood flow promoting herbs would. (This explains why one should not be on other blood flow promoting herbs for a long period of time.) *Sanqi* is also an ingredient in the commonly known prescription *yunnan baiyao* (云南白药) which is used for treating injuries due to trauma.

8.1.8 *Herbs for resolving phlegm* (化痰药)

Herbs for resolving phlegm, relieving cough and dyspnea, meaning difficulty in breathing, are further classified into two categories: herbs for resolving heat-phlegm and herbs for resolving wet-phlegm.

An example of a herb for resolving heat phlegm is *beimu* (贝母), which comes in two forms: *zhebeimu* (浙贝母) and *chuanbeimu* (川贝母). Between these two, *zhebeimu* is cooler and has a stronger effect in clearing heat phlegm and treating cough arising from heat syndrome. *Chuanbeimu*, on the other hand, has a stronger effect in moisturizing the lung even though it also helps to clear heat and resolve phlegm. Due to the slight differences in their properties, *zhebeimu* is often the choice for cough with viscous yellow phlegm whereas *chuanbeimu* is mostly used for treating chronic dry cough with little yellowish/ whitish phlegm, and it is the ingredient found in the popular cough syrup *chuanbeipipagao* (川贝枇杷膏).

A common herb for resolving wet phlegm is *banxia* (半夏), which is used together with *chenpi* in the formulation *erchentang* (二陈汤) to treat cough with wet phlegm and dampness. *Banxia* also removes dampness and disperses abnormal mass which helps to relieve abdominal distention. Another popular use of *banxia* by physicians is to relieve nausea and vomiting by suppressing adverse rise of stomach *qi*. Unprocessed *banxia* is toxic and in the past had to used with raw ginger to reduce its toxicity. Today, this does not pose a problem as *banxia* would have already undergone processing to reduce or remove its toxicity before distribution to medical halls.

Xingren (杏仁) or Chinese almonds are normally used for its cough relieving action, and it can be used to treat all types of cough because of its neutral nature. In addition, almond helps to moisten the large intestine to promote bowel movement because of its high oil content. There are two types of almonds, the northern and the southern almond. For the medicinal purposes and stronger therapeutic effects, northern almond, also known as bitter almond (*ku xingren*), would be the preferred choice as it relieves cough and dyspnea by promoting the descent of lung *qi*. Southern almonds, on the other hand, are often used for cooking and as snacks as they are sweeter and tastier, but their cough relieving action is much milder. Northern almonds are slightly toxic and should not be consumed in large quanitity.

8.1.9 *Tonics* (补益药)

TCM tonics or "restoratives for reinforcing asthenia"(补虚药, 补益药）are medicinal herbs for replenishing *qi*, blood, nourishing *yin* and *yang*, improving the functions of internal organs and body resistance to illness, and relieving the various kinds of symptoms of weakness. They are mostly sweet in flavour and warm in nature (except generally for *yin* tonics which tend to be cooling), which contributes to their nourishing and replenishing effects. Some rules regarding the use of tonics should be observed:

1. We should always differentiate what kind of deficiency syndromes one is having before taking tonics. Each category of tonic is used to address a different kind of deficiency syndrome. For example, *danggui* (当归) should be used in blood deficiency syndrome and not *yang* deficiency syndrome; ginseng should be used for either *qi* or *yang* deficiency syndrome and not on *yin* deficiency syndrome.
2. Do not use tonics when pathogens are active as that can aggravate the condition.
3. Tonics are more effective taken in small amounts over long periods of time. Excessive or wrong use of tonics can cause more harm to the body.
4. Many tonics are difficult to digest, hence it is generally advisable to mix tonics with herbs such as *shanyao* (山药) for strengthening the *qi* of the stomach and spleen and *chenpi* for regulating (improving the flow of) *qi*.

Qi Tonics (补气药)

These are mainly attributed to the spleen and lung meridians since lung dominates *qi* and the spleen is the main source for *qi* production hence promoting the functions of lung and spleen helps to replenish *qi*.

Ginseng (*renshen* 人参) is well known for its *qi*-tonifying action which makes one feel more energetic. It not only invigorates *qi* (大补元气) but also boosts *yang*. Among different types of ginseng, wild ginseng has the strongest effect in tonifying *qi* and is sometimes used in emergency life-threatening conditions when the patient is extremely weak from *qi* exhaustion.

Dangshen (党参), is also known as the 'the poor man's ginseng' because it is much less costly than *renshen*. *Dangshen* is weaker than ginseng as a *qi* tonic and is suitable for replenishing spleen *qi* and often used for long term chronic illnesses. *Taizishen* (太子参) replenishes spleen *qi* and promotes production of fluids to moisten the lung. Its therapeutic actions are milder as compared to those of *dangshen*.

American ginseng (*xiyangshen* 西洋参), also known as *huaqishen* (花旗参), is a different herb from (Chinese) ginseng. In Chinese terminology, it is not regarded as a form of ginseng, hence its Chinese name *xiyangshen* indicates it is a kind of root grown in America. Hence in English translation, to avoid confusion, when we refer to ginseng, we mean *renshen*. *Xiyangshen* is cool in nature, hence it is one of the few *qi* tonics that also have the action of clearing heat. It also promotes production of fluids and replenishes *qi* and *yin* and is therefore suitable for *qi* and *yin* deficiency of spleen and lung. *Xiyangshen* may be more suitable for people who live in tropical climates and enjoy rich and strongly-flavoured foods that tend to produce heat.

Another more common *qi* tonic used as food is Chinese yam (*shanyao* 山药). It is neutral and can be used in most people, whether young or elderly, because its therapeutic effects are mild. It nourishes not only the spleen/stomach and lung but also the kidney. It is considered a mild tonic for the spleen, lung and kidney, and can be taken for a long period of time, in both the fresh form as well as the dried medicinal form.

Yang Tonics (补阳药)

These are mainly attributed to the kidney meridian as the kidney is the main source of body *yang*. These herbs are used to treat kidney *yang* deficiency syndrome which is manifested as cold limbs, backaches, and sexual dysfunction; they are mostly sweet, pungent and salty in flavour and warm in nature. Cordyceps (*dongcongxiacao* 冬虫夏草) is a good tonic for strengthening lung *qi*. It strengthens the lung by boosting its *yang*, and tonifies kidney *yang*. As such, cordyceps are good for treating chronic cough due to weak lung and kidney functions.

Another example of *yang* tonic is *duzhong* (杜仲), which is a tree bark. It tonifies the kidney and liver and by doing so, it helps to strengthen the tendons and bones of the body. Often, it is used to treat backaches or body aches resulted from kidney and liver deficiency. It also helps maintain pregnancy by stabilizing the uterus.

Blood Tonics (补血药)

These are mainly attributed to the heart and liver meridians because heart governs blood and the liver stores blood. They are used to treat blood deficiency syndrome manifested as pale complexion, lip and nails, dizziness, palpitations, delayed menstruation, and insomnia. Two commonly used blood tonics are Chinese angelica (*danggui* 当归) and longan meat (*longyanrou* 龙眼肉).

Besides its blood nourishing action, Chinese angelica also has a mild blood flow promoting action, which explains why it can be used for relieving pain. Different part of Chinese angelica has different emphasis on its actions: the head has a stronger effect in nourishing blood whereas the tail is better used for promoting blood flow. In addition, Chinese angelica can also be used for treating constipation due to blood deficiency syndrome as it helps to moisten the large intestine to promote bowel movement by tonifying the blood. Although both nourish blood, Chinese angelica is usually used for regulating menstruation whereas longan meat is used for treating insomnia or palpitation arising from heart-blood deficiency syndrome. Longan meat strengthens the function of the heart and spleen through nourishing blood, which in turn helps to calm the mind for better sleep quality. In comparison, longan meat has a sweeter and pleasant taste than Chinese angelica, hence, it is a more popular choice for making tonic teas.

Yin Tonics (补阴药)

These are mainly attributed to the kidney, liver, lung and stomach meridians, and most of them are slightly cool in nature because *yin* deficiency syndromes usually come with heat symptoms due to asthenic fire. Symptoms manifested in *yin* deficiency syndromes are dryness in the mouth, throat and skin, hot flashes, tinnitus, soreness in the lower back, frequent hunger pangs with no weight gain, and a red tongue with thin fur.

Wolfberry (*gouqizi* 枸杞子) is a *yin* tonic which nourishes kidney and liver *yin*. Through this action, it helps to tonify *jing* (essence) and improves vision, especially for those who have dry eyes or redness of eyes due to kidney/liver yin deficiency. It is neutral in nature and can be used as food or medicine for most body constitutions. It is also believed that wolfberry helps to boost the immune system, and is useful for those who have undergone chemotherapy that weakens their immune system.

Lily bulb (*baihe* 百合) is also another *yin* tonic that is also used as food. It is cool in nature which clears asthenic (deficiency) heat from the heart to calm the mind; hence it can be used to treat insomnia due to heart *yin* deficiency syndrome. Lily bulb is also used to treat dry cough due to lung *yin* deficiency by nourishing and moistening the lung. Its nourishing *yin* action is stronger if it is processed with honey through baking. Although its property is mildly cool, it generally does not upset the digestive system and is suitable to most people, but its therapeutic actions are not very strong.

8.2 Medical Formulations (Prescriptions) (方剂)

Fangji (方剂) is the TCM term for a medical formulation or prescription. It is called a prescription because it is normally used for medical purposes by physicians, and not just a formulation for cooking herbal dishes or as a tasty tea drunk for prophylactic purposes. The word *fang* (方) means 'method'; in ordinary language, *youfang* (有方) means having the right method, or the correct approach to solving a problem; *ji* (剂) denotes a medical preparation. Hence *fangji* denotes medicine formulated by a good method, i.e. a well-formulated prescription.

Chinese physicians have found over the years that herbs can be combined in a certain way to achieve the best desired result, much as a cocktail drink has a clever combination of ingredients to yield a desired taste, or a food recipe to make an appetizing and nutritious dish. Unlike Western medicine, Chinese prescriptions are customised for the individual, taking into account the type and severity of his syndromes as well as his constitution and state of health.

However, Chinese medicine has over thousands of years also developed a large number of standard classical prescriptions that can be used as a base for patients falling within a category of syndromes. In practice, these prescriptions are often modified by the physician to suit the individual by taking out and/or adding some ingredients.

These standard prescriptions are classified by therapeutic effect, as for single herbs. Because the prescriptions contain several herbs, each playing a different role, a better result can usually be obtained than by using just one herb. This is in contrast to the typical Western drug which generally contains one active chemical ingredient with other ingredients only providing a non-active base for the delivery of the active ingredient. To deal with several conditions present together, a number of different drugs have to be taken simultaneously, in contrast to the Chinese approach in which the customised prescription treats one or more syndromes with one formulation.

8.2.1 *Preparing a decoction*

Chinese medicine prescriptions can come in many forms. The most common form familiar to most people is the decoction in which the herbs have to undergo an hour or so of boiling, sometimes longer, to extract the useful ingredients. The typical correct way to prepare the decoction is described as follow:

1. Soak the herbs in water for 20 minutes. There should be enough water to cover all the herbs.
2. Bring the herbs to boil and continue cooking with low heat for another 45 minutes. Decant.
3. Add water into the pot of herbs and bring it to boil. After boiling, use low heat for another 30 minutes. Decant.
4. Mix the first and second bowls to achieve an even concentration of the decoction as the first bowl would have been more concentrated than the second.
5. After mixing, divide the decoction into two separate bowls and one bowl can be kept in the refrigerator for later consumption. Drink the decoction warm.

8.2.2 *Other forms of prescriptions*

Other forms of prescriptions include powder, pill, honeyed boluses, concentrated pills, special pills and medicated wine.

Honeyed boluses are much bigger than pills/concentrated pills and special pills; they have to be bitten to break into smaller pieces before chewing and swallowing. These two forms of prescriptions are usually given for chronic illnesses and taken over a longer period of time.

Medicated wine basically is herbs soaked in strong wine, usually one of the Chinese white wines like *gaoliang* (高粱). Soaking the herbs in wine enables its useful ingredients to be extracted, while at the same time boosting the therapeutic actions of the herbs. Such wines should be taken in smaller amount each time since their therapeutic effects are much stronger.

In modern times, with better processing technology and consumer demand for more convenient ways to take their medications, the forms of prescription commonly used in many TCM clinics are powders, liquids or capsules/tablets that have been prepared by extraction techniques and presented in hygienic packaging.

8.2.3 *The art and science of combining herbs*

The general principle for combining herbs for a TCM prescription is based on the concept of each of the herbs playing one of four possible roles such that in combination they have the most desirable effect: a sort of team combination. The roles have colourful names, related to hierarchies in Chinese emperor's courts. They are known as the monarch, ministerial, adjuvant and guiding roles, as the Chinese terms being *jun* (君), *chen* (臣), *zuo* (佐), *shi* (使), respectively.

1. The Monarch or *jun* herb plays the core therapeutic role as it targets the main syndrome.
2. The Ministerial or *chen* herb enhances the monarch's effect.

3. The Adjuvant or *zuo* herb plays a complementary role, supporting the monarch or/and minister herb by working on a related concomitant condition, or reducing toxicities and side effects, if any, of the monarch and ministerial herbs.
4. The Guiding or *shi* herb helps direct the other herbs to the particular organs and harmonises their joint action.

It is not necessary for every formulation to embody all four roles, although almost all formulations would have at least two to three of these roles covered by the constituent herbs. Of course, the simplest formulation of all is the single herb. For example, the ginseng decoction *dushentang* (独参汤), which only contains ginseng plays the monarch role by invigorating *qi* in the body. This formulation is sometimes used to treat life-threatening conditions in which the person is critically ill and very weak; the dosage of ginseng used is relatively high.

It is also not always the case that there is only one herb for each role. Often, there are several herbs playing the same role each in its own way because of its particular flavour and properties. We shall see examples of these when we examine some classical formulations.

We cover only some basic formulations below, with explanations on their compositions. More formulations and their clinical applications and therapeutic actions are summarised in Annex 2.

8.2.4 Some classical formulations that have stood the test of time

Decoction of the Four Noble Herbs
(Sijunzi Tang 四君子汤)

This is a formulation for tonifying *qi* and treating *qi* deficiency syndrome of spleen. It replenishes *qi* and also strengthens the spleen functions. It comprises four herbs; with ginseng (人参) as the monarch herb, *baizhu* (白术) as the minister herb, *fuling* (茯苓) as the adjuvant herb and *zhigancao* (炙甘草) as the guiding herb. Ginseng is a *qi* tonic and it targets the main syndrome by boosting the level of *qi* in the body. *Baizhu* enhances the action of replenishing *qi* and at the same time strengthens the spleen functions by removing dampness which often accompanies weakness of the spleen and stomach. *Fuling* plays the complementary role of strengthening the therapeutic actions of both ginseng and *baizhu*. *Zhigancao* completes the picture, harmonising the actions of the other herbs; in itself it is also a mild spleen-*qi* tonic.

Extensions: This formulation can be extended for the same family of ailments but with different therapeutic emphasis. For example, adding *chenpi* (陈皮) and *banxia* (半夏) to the formulation creates the Decoction of the Six Noble Herbs (*Liujunzi Tang* 六君子汤) which addresses spleen deficiency with dampness and phlegm characterised by poor appetite, loose stools, nausea, wet phlegm and thick or greasy white fur. The presence of dampness and phlegm is more pronounced in this syndrome, which explains the addition of *chenpi* and *banxia* to resolve the dampness and phlegm.

When dampness and phlegm have affected the flow of *qi* in the spleen in the patient, manifested in abdominal distension with frequent flatulence, *qi*-regulating herbs such as *muxiang* (木香) and *sharen* (砂仁) can be further added to remove *qi* stagnation and restore *qi* flow in the spleen. This yields *Xiangsha Liujunzi Tang* (香砂六君子汤).

Decoction of the Four Ingredients (*Siwu Tang* 四物汤)

This is a basic formulation for tonifying blood and is used to treat the blood deficiency syndrome. It is composed of *shuihuang* (熟地黄) (monarch), *danggui* (当归) (minister);

chuanxiong (川芎) and *baishao* (白芍) together play the adjuvant role. *Shudihuang*, *danggui* and *baishao* nourish blood whereas *chuanxiong* promotes the blood flow so that the whole combination has the overall effect of nourishing and regulating blood without introducing stasis. This formulation can be used for regulating menstruation, and can also be given after menstruation.

Extensions: When there is also blood deficiency with blood stasis, two blood promoting herbs *taoren* (桃仁) and *honghua* (红花) are added and the resulting formulation *Taohong Siwu Tang* (桃红四物汤) has a stronger effect of promoting blood flow and removing stasis.

Combining the Decoction of the Four Noble Herbs and the Decoction of the Four Ingredients gives us the popular formulation Decoction of 8 Precious Ingredients (*Bazhen Tang* 八珍汤), much loved by housewives who buy them from medical halls as well as grocery stores. This decoction addresses both *qi* and blood deficiency syndromes. The monarch herbs are ginseng and *shudihuang*, with the principal effect of nourishing both *qi* and blood. *Bazhen Tang* is normally used for prolonged weakness of *qi* and blood caused by excessive hemorrhage and depletion of *qi*. Because this formulation is warm in nature and has strong tonic properties, it should be taken in moderation, preferably with medical advice.

Pill of Six Ingredients with Rehmanniae (Liuwei Dihuang Wan 六味地黄丸)

This is a basic formulation for nourishing *yin* and is used in the deficiency syndrome of kidney and liver *yin* which leads to a flare up of kidney deficiency fire. The symptoms are tinnitus, night sweat, emission, sore throat. This syndrome is often seen in menopausal and post-menopausal women as well as diabetic patients.

It consists of three tonics and three purgatives. The three tonics are *shudihuang* (熟地黄) (monarch), *shanzhuyu* (山茱萸) and *shanyao* (山药) (both are ministers); *fuling* (茯苓), *mudanpi* (牡丹皮) and *zexie* (泽泻), all of which play the primary adjuvant role of purging heat. There is no guiding herb. *Shudihuang* nourishes kidney *yin* and essence; *shanzhuyu* enhances the action of nourishing kidney and liver *yin*; *shanyao* strengthens spleen and reinforces the action of nourishing the kidney. The three adjuvant herbs play varying roles of reducing dampness, clearing heat arising from *yin* deficiency and improving the transportation and transformation function of the spleen. This is appropriate since the health of the kidney is strongly dependent on the healthy functioning of the spleen to provide nutrients to the vital organs, including the kidney, to sustain body activities.

Liuwei Dihuang Wan tonifies the kidney and spleen as well as dissipates internal heat in a balanced and gentle manner, making it one of the most successful prescriptions in the history of Chinese medicine. It is used equally by physicians treating illnesses, as well as by the common man as a dietary supplement to combat the weakening of the kidney functions that comes with stress and ageing.

Extensions: For strengthening kidney *yang* rather than *yin*, two warm herbs can be added to turn *Liuwei Dihuang Wan* into another classic formulation called the Pill for Nourishing Kidney *Yang* (*Shenqi wan* 肾气丸). The herbs *guizhi* (桂枝) and *fuzi* (附子) warm and invigorate the kidney. As the therapeutic emphasis of the formulation has changed from nourishing *yin* to warming *yang*, the monarch herbs are now *guizhi* and *fuzi*, with *shudihuang* as the minister herb.

Another variation of this formulation is used in cases in which the deficiency of kidney *yang* has worsened and led to water retention, diuretics such as *chuanniuxi* (川牛膝) and *cheqianzi* (车前子) are added to form the formulation *Jisheng*

Shenqi Wan (济生肾气丸) giving it the ability to aid in removing excess water from the body through urination. This formulation is also used by some physicians for treating urination problems due to benign prostate enlargement.

Erchen Tang (二陈汤)

This is a basic formulation for treating wet phlegm and is often used in wet cough due to phlegm-dampness syndrome with white sputum. *Banxia* (半夏) is the monarch herb and it targets the main syndrome by resolving phlegm and dampness. *Chenpi* (陈皮), the minister herb, enhances the action of *banxia* to remove phlegm and dampness; it helps to regulate spleen *qi* since the presence of dampness and phlegm in the body tends to result in *qi* stagnation. *Fuling* (茯苓), which is the adjuvant, strengthens the action of removing dampness through the promotion of urination, and itself is also a mild spleen tonic. *Zhigancao* (炙甘草), the guiding herb, helps to harmonise the therapeutic actions of the herbs in the formulation. The overall therapeutic action is to dry dampness, resolve phlegm and promote *qi* flow.

"Ease" Powder (Xiaoyao San 逍遥散)

The name of this formulation actually already tells you what it might be used for. The renowned ancient Taoist philosopher Zhuangzi in his celebrated essay *Xiaoyao You* (逍遥游) describes a mythical giant roc that flies at the speed of sound, cruising at ease without a care in the world. The 'ease' powder formulation borrows its name from the legend, and is usually prescribed to individuals who suffer from stagnation of liver *qi* and deficiency of blood and spleen syndrome because of stress and anxiety that affect the smooth flow of the liver *qi* and leads to liver *qi* stagnation, which in turn suppresses the spleen function.

Individuals who exhibit this syndrome besides having moodiness, headache, irregular menstruation, and a taut pulse also present symptoms associated with weak spleen functions like poor appetite, lassitude and loose stools. This complex formulation contains, among others, *chaihu* (柴胡) (monarch), which disperses liver-*qi* stagnation, *Baishao* (白芍) and *danggui* (当归) (ministers) which nourish liver blood to sustain the liver *qi*-dredging function, with *fuling* (茯苓), *baizhu* (白术) and *zhigancao* (炙甘草) as adjuvants aiding *qi* and fortifying the spleen against liver repression. *Zhigancao* is used as a guiding herb playing a harmonising role.

If the syndrome progresses further and the patient develops fire resulting from prolonged stagnation of liver *qi*, *mudanpi* (牡丹皮) and *zhizi* (栀子) are added to form *Danzhi Xiaoyaosan* (丹栀逍遥散), which has the additional function of purging liver fire which is commonly manifested by symptoms of a fiery temper, red eyes, and vexatiousness.

Jade-screen Powder (Yupingfeng San 玉屏风散)

This formulation addresses deficiency in defensive-*qi* syndrome which is characterised by profuse perspiration with aversion to wind, pale complexion, and susceptibility to the invasion of exogenous climatic pathogens especially wind. Its main therapeutic action is to replenish *qi* especially in the strengthening of defensive *qi* and arresting perspiration. Individuals who have this syndrome tend to have low *zhengqi* and to catch colds or flu more easily.

Huangqi (黄芪) is the monarch herb, replenishing *qi* and consolidating the outer layer of the body (superficies) so that the body is not vulnerable to the invasion of the exogenous pathogens. *Baizhu* (白术) further enhances the action of tonifying *qi* by strengthening the spleen as it is the source of *qi* and blood production; *fangfeng* (防风) assists in the building up of body resistance by expelling exogenous wind pathogens.

Pulse-activating Powder (Shengmai Yin 生脉饮)

Playing a different role from Jade-screen powder, this formulation is used to treat spontaneous sweating arising from the presence of both *qi* and *yin* deficiency syndrome. It is also used in the treatment of chronic dry cough accompanied by breathlessness, fatigue, dryness in throat and profuse sweating. Ginseng, the monarch herb, addresses *qi* deficiency whereas the minister herb *maidong* (麦冬) helps to resolve *yin* deficiency by nourishing *yin* to moisten the lung. *Wuweizi* (五味子), the adjuvant herb, helps in the production of fluids and arrests sweating so as to prevent excessive loss of body fluids which would further exacerbate *yin* deficiency.

Shengmai Yin can be prescribed to persons subjected to prolonged hot weather causing excessive perspiration and damage to the *yin* of the body and depleting its reserves of *qi*.

9

Navigating the Body's Meridian Network

Acupuncture and Tuina

During Richard Nixon's historic visit to China in 1972, his entourage witnessed one of the wonders of ancient Chinese science in action. Brain surgery was conducted with the patient fully awake, and a woman after delivery by a Caesarean operation while fully conscious got up from the operating table and walked to the recovery bed. All this took place with acupuncture needles placed in strategic points on the patients' bodies. Western expert opinions vary as to whether the patients received painkillers and other drugs during those procedures, but there was no doubt that acupuncture needles played a key anaesthetic role.

The drama of these procedures was not lost on the American television audience, and interest in this ancient science surged in the West. Today acupuncture is practised in the United States with licensing boards for practitioners and eligibility for medical insurance claims in most states. It is used mainly to treat pain, although trained practitioners can treat a variety of conditions with acupuncture techniques.

9.1 History of Acupuncture

Acupuncture as a tool for healing likely predated the use of herbs. In the Stone Age knives and needles were carved from stones and bones to prick the body, draw blood or lance abscesses. During the Warring States period (475–221 BC) metal needles replaced sharpened stones, as suggested by archaeological findings in 1968 of the nine metal needles (five silver and four gold needles) recorded in the *Huangdi Neijing* for acupuncture.

The theory of acupuncture and meridian system was extensively documented in the *Neijing* in which 160 acupuncture points identified. The number of points was increased to 349 in the *Systemic Classics of Acupuncture and Moxibustion* (*Zhenjiu Jia Yi Jing*).

Over the years, much advancement has been made in the techniques of acupuncture and, together with the development of fine sterile filiform needles used today, acupuncture has gradually been systematised as a scientific procedure, studied in universities and research centers as an important discipline within Chinese medicine.

The Chinese term for acupuncture is commonly used to mean *zhenjiu* (针灸), which actually embodies two related modes of therapy, namely acupuncture (*zhen* 针) and moxibustion (*jiu* 灸). To avoid confusion, in this chapter we use acupuncture to mean the former, which employs thin metal needles to penetrate the skin so as to stimulate the acupuncture point, creating a sore and numb sensation. This can be done manually or by connecting the needle to a device that generates electric pulses. Moxibustion uses moxa floss processed from mugwort leaves in tube or fusiform shape, with one end smoking and placed it above an acupuncture point or over a body area. Moxibustion warms the body to improve the flows of *qi* and blood. It is sometimes combined with acupuncture to enhance their effects.

9.2 The Meridian System

The underlying principle of acupuncture as for other modalities of Chinese medicine is to regulate *yin* and *yang* to restore balance and stimulate the flow of *qi* and blood. Moxibustion's main effect is to warm the channels, disperse cold pathogens and resolve blood stasis and stagnation.

The 'meridian system' (*jingluo* 经络) forms the diagnosis and treatment framework for acupuncture and moxibustion, as well as for *tuina*, which we shall cover later in this chapter. In TCM theory, the meridian system is a network of passages that transports *qi*, blood, *jing*, *yin* and *yang* throughout the body, connecting vital organs and linking all other parts of the body including the bone, skin, muscles and tendons and the nine orifices, thus allowing the body to function as an organic whole. The system also maintains communication between the body and its external environment to help achieve a balance between the body and its host environment. The meridian system is therefore much more than a neurological network, but a much bigger system with functions so broad as to rival those of the organ system.

The term 'meridian' is used in two ways in TCM theory. It could refer to the entire system, or to the main trunk routes in the system; the context of use usually makes it clear which is being referred to. The meridian system (*jingluo* 经络) comprises main trunk routes, the meridians (*jing* 经) and smaller branches called collaterals (*luo* 络) that criss-cross to form an intricate network. The meridians run at the level of muscles and organs and hence are at a deeper level than the collaterals, which mostly run at the level of or just below the skin. All the meridians run vertically, with the exception of the *dai* (带) meridian which runs transversely around the body.

The meridians in TCM are analogous to roads and highways that link villages, cities, farms, and industrial installations in a country. They contain *qi* and can become diseased when invaded by pathogens, or they can develop obstructions that hinder the flow of *qi* and communication signals along them. The meridians therefore behave as if they were a parallel set of organs so that by one method of TCM disease analysis, specific meridian-based pathological conditions can be identified.

The principal components of the network are the 12 main meridians (*jingmai* 经脉) and eight 'extraordinary vessels' (*qijing bamai* 奇经八脉). Each of the 12 main meridians is connected to a particular organ and is named after that organ. Hence on speaks of the spleen meridian, the bladder meridian, and the like. The five ordinary *zang* organs together with pericardium make up six *zang* organs matching six *fu* organs, each of which could be connected to the 12 main meridians.

The six meridians associated with the *zang*-organs are deemed to be *yin* in nature, and the others associated with the *fu*-organs *yang* in nature. These classifications reflect the

Chinese propensity for balance and symmetry. Among other things, the *yang* meridians run along those parts of the body that face the sun (the back and the outside of the limbs), while the *yin* meridians are on the chest and the inside of the limbs, which are usually shaded from the sun. The meridian associated with the triple burner (*sanjiao* 三焦) *fu*-organ is paired with the pericardium meridian.

The eight 'extraordinary vessels' have no direct connection to the *zang* and *fu*-organs. The most commonly used extraordinary vessels for therapy, particularly acupuncture therapy, are the governor vessel (*dumai* 督脉), the conception vessel (*renmai* 任脉), and the thorough fare vessel (*chongmai* 冲脉). The *dumai* is thought to 'govern' the *yang* meridians and the *renmai* the *yin* meridians. The *chongmai* is termed 'the sea of blood' as it is deemed to be the place where all *qi* and blood in the body converge.

The relevance of the meridians in TCM goes far beyond therapy for pain. Their main use lies in their association with and connection to particular organs. For example, acupuncture needles applied to points along the spleen and stomach meridians can have a tonifying effect on these organs, hence they are often used for patients with digestive disorders. Acupuncture can also be applied to certain points to dissipate internal heat. Acupuncture of points along the *renmai* and *chongmai* are used to treat gynaecological problems as there is thought to be a connection of these extraordinary vessels to the uterus.

9.3 Tuina

Tuina employs the same therapeutic principles as acupuncture which is to regulate *yin* and *yang*, achieve harmony and balance in the body and stimulate smooth flow of *qi* and blood by working on the meridians and acupuncture points. Instead of using fine needles to stimulate the acupuncture points, *tuina* adopts a non-invasive method by applying pressure on the points and/or the meridians.

It is important to note that *tuina* is different from ordinary massage practised in health spas. *Tuina* applies TCM theory for therapeutic effects on pain and such conditions as digestive and menstruation disorders, and insomnia.

Child *tuina* can be performed on children including infants for which its therapeutic functions include enhancing the child's health by boosting the functions of the organs, especially respiratory and digestive systems, promoting overall growth and development and strengthening bonding with parents and children. It is believed that regular *tuina* helps to strengthen the child's immune system and well-being.

As for adult *tuina*, child *tuina* also requires the application of pressure, with less force, on the acupuncture points. A child's acupuncture points are usually not as sharply defined, and come in the form of area or zone rather than a small point. For instance, rubbing the first segment of the child's thumb is equivalent to pressing the acupuncture point *zusanli* (足三里) on the spleen meridian, and both have the same effect of strengthening the spleen functions. Lubricants such as talcum powder or baby's oil are necessary in child *tuina* to reduce the friction. The choice of acupuncture points and techniques depends on the age, body constitution and underlying syndrome of the patient; this applies equally to adult and child *tuina*.

9.4 Acupuncture Points

There are a total of 361 acupuncture points recorded to date and each of them has its own specific set of clinical applications. Application of needles or acupressure on the points can have the effect of tonifying, regulating *qi* and blood flow, promoting balance and removing heat or warming action, depending on the techniques and manipulation methods used.

According to the characteristics of the acupuncture points, they can be classified into three categories:

1) Meridian points (*jingxue* 经穴) are found along the 12 main meridians, governor vessel and conception vessel (a total of 14 meridians). These points have fixed locations and their clinical applications are closely related to their corresponding meridians. For example, most of the points on the conception vessel are used to treat gynaecological problems; and the points on the kidney meridian mostly have therapeutic effects of strengthening the kidney functions.

2) Extraordinary points (*qixue* 奇穴) are not located on the 14 meridians. For example, the point *taiyang* (太阳), which resides at our temple is used in ailments such as headache, eye disorders and facial paralysis. In general, the extraordinary points have narrower clinical applications.

3) *Ashi* points (*ashixue* 阿是穴) are tender spots that are not marked by fixed location and do not have any direct relationship with any of the meridians. They do not have a specific name and are generally known as the *ashi* points. They are used mainly in pain treatments as they are located by the physicians based on the area where it is most painful.

Among the acupuncture points used in TCM, there are some common points which are convenient for applying pressure ourselves on a daily basis to promote health. Some common ones are described below.

Hegu (合谷)

Location: It is situated at the back of the hand, between the first and second metacarpal.

Applications: Pain in facial region (example, headache, toothache, sore eyes etc); external syndrome of coughs and colds. Pregnant women should avoid pressing it.

Neiguan (内关)

Location: It is situated three fingers up from the inner side of the wrist, between the two tendons.

Applications: Heart problems such as mild angina pain, heart palpitation; digestive disorders such as gastric pain, nausea, vomiting; dizziness, car sickness, migraine; insomnia, depression, stroke, tightness in the chest.

Zusanli (足三里)

Location: It is situated four fingers down from the center of the depression on the outer side of the knee cap.

Applications: Digestive problems and it is good for improving general well-being.

Taiyang (太阳)

Location: It is situated at the head region, one middle finger away from the temple.

Applications: Migrane, headache, eye disorders, facial paralysis

Baihui (百会)

Location: At the head region. It is the midpoint of the line joining the tips of the ears.

Applications: Headache, insomnia, stroke, forgetfulness, dizziness.

Shuigou (水沟) [*also known as renzhong* (人中)]

Location: At the face region. It is situated on the upper one-third of the philtrum which is the area between the nose and the upper lip.

Applications: It is often used during emergencies such as fainting, unconsciousness, stroke and epilepsy; it also helps nasal congestion.

Fengchi (风池)

Location: It is the depression found at the back of the neck below the occipital which is the base of the skull.

Applications: Neck stiffness; internal wind syndromes that result in stroke, epilepsy, dizziness; external wind syndromes that result in colds and nasal congestion. The main therapeutic effect of *fengchi* is to expel wind pathogens.

Guanyuan (关元)

Location: It is situated four fingers down from the navel.

Applications: Gynecological and andrological disorders; urinary tract disorders; abdominal pain, diarrhea, dysentery, sterility, prolapse of rectum, other intestinal disorders; deficiency due to cold and exhaustion; other conditions due to deficiency of original *qi*. It has the therapeutic effect of warming the body.

Sanyinjiao (三阴交)

Location: It is situated four fingers up from the ankle bone protrusion, at the inner part of the leg.

Applications: Digestive disorders; gynecological problems; urinary problems; *yin* deficiency syndromes. Pregnant women should avoid pressing it.

Taichong (太冲)

Location: It is situated at the back of the feet, between the first and second metatarsus.

Applications: Syndromes arise from liver imbalances (liver heat, liver *yin* deficiency etc) that result in headache, dizziness, eye redness, gynecological problems (irregular menses, menstruation cramps, heavy flow).

Among the above commonly-used points, it has been suggested that the first three Zusanli, Hegu and Neiguan, would most benefit health and disease prevention. Acupressure using fingers or a short stick with a rounded end for 15 minutes on each of these points, done two to three times a day, can go some way to strengthen *qi*, improve flows in the body, strengthen the heart and improve mental agility.

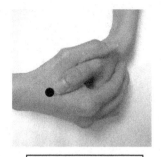

合谷 Hegu

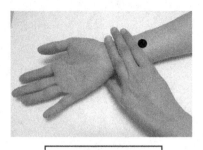

内关 Neiguan

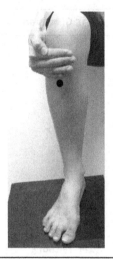

足三里 Zusanli

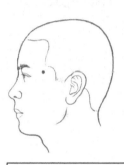

太阳 Taiyang

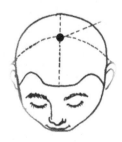

百会 Baihui

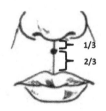

水沟 Shuigou

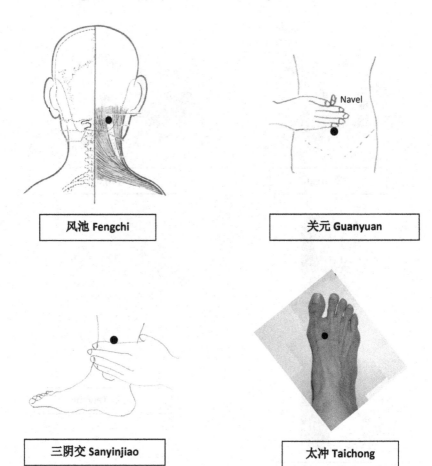

风池 Fengchi

关元 Guanyuan

Navel

三阴交 Sanyinjiao

太冲 Taichong

10

Attaining Longevity and Vitality

The art and science of cultivating life

In Chapter 6 we caught a glimpse of the broad principles of the ancients in cultivating good health and avoiding illness. We now look at the subsequent development of these basic ideas over the centuries and how modern knowledge of physiology and nutrition can be incorporated to provide us with practical guidelines for good health.

On the broader human landscape, the Chinese tradition of *yangsheng* is not just about achieving health, but a complete culture of finding spiritual fulfilment and happiness which are deeply intertwined with attaining a healthy mind and body. In the Chinese word for *yangsheng*, the word *yang* (养) means cultivate, and *sheng* (生) means life. *Yangsheng* then is more than the cultivation of health: it is the cultivation of life itself.

10.1 Aspects of *Yangsheng*

We may break down *yangsheng* into its many facets. These include:

yangshen	养身	cultivating the body
yangxin	养心	cultivating calm and tranquility
yangxing	养性	cultivating one's character
yangshen	养神	cultivating the spirit

In some ways, the pecking order in the above list reflects the difficulty of each level of cultivation. Cultivating the body is the easiest, and attaining a cultivated spirit is the hardest and most elusive.

Cultivating the body or *yangshen* (养身) involves appropriate nutrition, regularity in living habits, and getting enough exercise, avoiding harmful environmental influences like harsh weather, and avoiding excesses of emotion like anger and anxiety.

Avoiding harmful pathogens mainly requires good hygiene, dressing appropriately for the seasons and the time of the day, and staying away from extreme cold, heat, dampness, dryness and wind.

To *yangxin* (养心) is cultivate calm and tranquillity. This requires both nurturing the physical health of our heart as an organ involved in calming the mind and promoting sleep, but also enjoying the soothing freshness and salubrious ambience of a nature walk, or relaxing by the cool waters of a stream, or watching the sun rise from the porch of your apartment. Many of the formulations in TCM have calming effects on the heart: foods like *lingzhi* and *baihe* also have calming effects. One formulation known as *Yangxin Tang* (养心汤) calms the nerves and fortifies the heart against shocks and irritations that may upset the person who has a weak heart.

The growing interest worldwide in mindfulness and meditation is a healthy trend, and reflects the need for people living in stressful environments to *yangxin*. Meditation has been shown since the 1960s to have salutary effects on our nervous systems, in particular the parasympathetic nervous system that employs neurotransmitters to make the body to cope with stress and calm the nerves. This in turn has beneficial effects on a broad range of conditions like hypertension, gastric disorders and cardiovascular disease.[14]

Cultivating character or *yangxing* (养性) is an important value in Chinese culture, emphasised particularly by Confucian ethics that stresses education and training from a young age to appreciate and practise the virtue of kindness and consideration for others, as well as the discipline of good manners and protocol (also known as *li* (礼) or 'rites' in Confucian ethics) that trains a person to control his temper and develop patience and determination in the conduct of his life.

The virtues of kindness and benevolence toward others may not appear to be much related to the health of the body, but modern psychologists are finding out what the ancients knew all along, that a kind and compassionate heart is good for health of mind and body. For example, Thupten Jinpa argues that a

---

[14] Herbert Benson and his colleagues at Harvard Medical School did extensive studies in the 1960s that established the scientific basis for the medical benefits of meditation. See Benson, H and Klipper, MZ (1975) *The Relaxation Response*. Mass Market Paperback.

compassionate heart over time can alter the physiology of our brains to make it more resilient and able to deal with anxiety and depression.[15] Being benevolent towards others helps contribute to one's feeling of self worth, imparts satisfaction of doing something useful and charitable for one's fellow men, and enhances our sense of self worth. Such an attitude of mind can be helpful toward our own emotional health.

Finally, *yangshen* (养神) or cultivation of the spirit is the hardest but most rewarding of all. Each person may have a different path to it. Some achieve it through religion and prayers, others through art and music, and yet others through a variety of creative activities that stimulate and bring out their deeper selves. The Taoist philosophers were among the masters of cultivating the spirit. The Chinese art of calligraphy and brush painting and the playing of musical instruments like the *qin*, and the appreciation and writing of poetry are activities that lift the human spirit to a level even beyond that of self-actualisation that stood at the apex of Maslow's famous pyramid of human needs. Various aspects of *yangsheng* were emphasised by ancient masters. We briefly look at three examples of these masters who came from varying periods of China's ancient history.

10.2 Ancient Masters of *Yangsheng*

Ji Kang (嵇康) (223–262 AD)

Ji Kang was brought up as a Confucian scholar who mastered the art of the *sanwen* (散文), a form of Chinese literature that uses eloquently-worded arguments in essays to expound new ideas, persuade the readers, or evoke strong feelings in them. He

---

[15] Jinpa, T (2015) *A Fearless Heart*. London: Piatkus (Little, Brown Book Group).

later converted to Taoism which people of his era found more comforting to the spirit as those were harsh times when violent despots ruled the land and life was brutal and uncertain. He became a member of a small group of Taoists who met regularly in a bamboo grove to write poetry, play music, enjoy wine and engage in intellectual and literary conversation. Known as "the seven sages of the bamboo grove", the group found a leader in the brilliant and charismatic Ji Kang.

Ji Kang, who was knowledgeable in Chinese medicine and practised it, emphasised the mind over body. His famous work was arguably *Yangsheng Lun* (养生论) which examined in depth the influence of the human mind and spirit on physical health. One of his famous lines was "The mind has sovereignty over the body: when the mind is disturbed, the body will be injured, as when an incompetent and self-indulgent ruler ruins a nation"(精神之于形骸,犹国之有君也;神躁于中,而形丧于外,犹君昏于上, 国乱与下也.) On the power of the mind over the body, he gave the example of how some patients treated with diaphoretic herbs to induce sweating do not respond yet, when frightened or anxious, break into profuse sweating. Another example was of the frail young girl whom tonic herbs failed to bring colour to her pale complexion, but a teasing word that embarrassed her turned her face crimson. Ji Kang was also a genius in musical composition. His love for music was expressed with his famous words, "I can live for a day without food, but not without music."

Ji Kang offended the emperor after he was summoned to serve in the imperial court but declined as he preferred the carefree life in his beloved Bamboo Grove, for which he was executed, leaving behind some of the best essays, poetry and musical works in Chinese history. But his legendary musical composition *Guanglinsan* (广陵散) that reputedly elevated the spirit to the heavenly sphere was lost forever, even though over the centuries many attempts were made by artists to re-create it from their own imaginations.

Zhu Danxi (朱丹溪) (1280–1358 AD)

Zhu Danxi, who lived in the Jin-Yuan dynasty period among the affluent gentry, observed that many people suffered from chronic disease mainly due to over-indulgence in rich food and sexual pleasures, and tended to suffer from an excess of *yang* and a deficiency in *yin*. Zhu postulated that nature and human lives are governed by movement and that all movements are based on 'ministerial fire' or *xianghuo* (相火) ("天主生物, 故恒于动; 人有此生, 亦恒于动。其所以恒于动, 皆相火之为也。")

Ministerial fire is a special term used in TCM to refer to the fire or *yangqi* originating from the 'life gate' (*mingmen* 命门) stored in the liver, gall bladder and the triple energiser in cooperation with heart *yang*. Access to the *mingmen* can be made through the *mingmen* acupuncture point located on the governor (*du*) meridian between the second and third lumbar verterbrae.[16] It reputedly warms and nourishes the vital organs and promotes their functions. Excessive ministerial fire results in damage of *yin*.

Zhu Danxi's *yangsheng* philosophy revolved around the dictum "There is excess of *yang*, and deficiency in *yin*" (阳有余, 阴不足). He strongly advocated nourishing *yin* to quench ministerial fire, and the nourishing of *yin* became the hallmark of his philosophy of *yangsheng*. Deficiency in *yin* was seen among the affluent and powerful who enjoyed life excessively.

---

[16] The notion of the *mingmen* in fact is somewhat obscure in TCM theory and several other versions of the *mingmen* exist in ancient literature, as is the exact location of the *mingmen* acupuncture point.

Such lifestyles are reminiscent of modern times in bustling cities of developed countries where over-indulgence results in diseases caused by *yin* deficiency, which could include diabetes, coronary heart disease, hypertension and certain cancers.

The remedy is to nourish *yin*, which can be achieved through dietary changes with the judicious use of *yin* tonics, particularly for the liver and kidney. In addition, mindfulness and slowing down of the pace of life can help to calm fire, and does regular *tuina* of the *du* meridian to release pent-up fire.

Wan Quan (万全) (1495–1585)

Wan Quan lived in the Ming dynasty in China, an era that saw the flowering of the arts and some of the most exquisite ceramic artifacts were made. Wan was a famed pediatrician who advocated that children be frequently exposed to sunlight and fresh air and trained to resist cold. He also believed that frightening a child was harmful, and discouraged over-feeding or excessive use of tonics and medications. In modern terms, we could interpret Wan Quan as believing in building up a person's immune system by natural means to form a strong foundation for his health through life.

For adults, Wan summarised his philosophy of *yangsheng* in four cardinal principles:

1. Living an ascetic lifestyle, free of desire (寡欲)
2. Preserving original *qi*, or *yuan qi* (慎动)
3. Regulating and balancing *yin yang* (法时)
4. Use natural means to prevent illness, and use prudence and caution in the use of herbal medicines (却疾)

The first three guidelines were elaborations and extensions of the ideas laid down by the *Neijing*. The fourth contains a useful warning against the use of medicines as a substitute for healthy diets and lifestyles. Wan pointed out that most medicines have toxic side effects to different degrees and should be avoided unless they are really needed. Wan's insight here could apply equally in modern times, cautioning us against the use of dietary supplements rather than eating wholesome meals with good quality ingredients. As Pollan and others point out, modern processed foods give us inadequate nutrition as essential vitamins and other components of food may have been destroyed or altered by processing, and we also do not always eat a balanced diet.[17] Hence there is a perceived need to use supplements to make up for deficiencies in the diet, but this requires expert knowledge on the use of these supplements in the right amounts and combinations. Nutrition specialists often point out the injudicious and excessive use of supplements may overall do more harm than good.

The same principle applies to the use of TCM tonics and medications. Without adequate knowledge or advice from a physician, it is common for people to take herbs that are not suitable for their conditions or constitutions, or simply take too much of them. Wan Quan's call for prudence in the use of medicines is appropriate for our times, even if his warnings were sounded more than 500 years ago.

10.3 Ageing and Longevity

Why do we age? Biologists tell us that human beings have built-in mechanisms for physiological processes to slowly decline as we get older. Much of it has to do with the ability of cells in the body to regenerate. Ageing is regulated by specific genes. Some cells continuously replicate *in vivo*, but have a finite replicative

---

[17] Pollan, M (2006) *The Omnivore's Dilemma.* Penguin.

life. The telomere at the end of a chromosome, which ensures cell replication, shortens as we age: each time a cell divides, some sequences of the telomere are lost; eventually, after about 60–100 divisions in an average cell, the cell dies.[18] Replication of telomeres is directed by the enzyme telomerase. Hence delaying the telomerase to some extent can be boosted by supplementing the body's telomerase. Drugs like resveratrol extracted from red wine, as well as Chinese herbs like *astragalus* (*huangqi*) can perform this function.

Other systems of the body also decline with age. The body's immune system undergoes age-dependent decline. Lymphocytes from older adults have less ability to multiply. The neurological system declines as neurons do not replicate and older ones die. These molecular mechanisms predispose older persons to dysfunction in the face of stress and disease. The result is impaired wound healing and increased risk of infection.[19]

These biological changes are accompanied by physiological declines. Cardiac output is reduced, the elasticity of lung decreases, there is a greater tendency to develop metabolic syndrome, fluid and electrolyte homeostasis are affected, and vision and hearing suffer neurological decline. Inflammation, the body's defense against invaders such as harmful bacteria, viruses, and toxins, involves oxidative stress, a biological rusting of our tissues and organs can further disrupt the immune system to accelerate ageing and the development of chronic illnesses like diabetes, arthritis and cardiovascular diseases.

It can thus be seen that to slow down ageing and achieve higher longevity, it is important to avoid stress and improper diet that lead to inflammation. Use of supplements that increase

---

[18] *Oxford Medical Dictionary*. Oxford (2007).

[19] Abrass, IB (1990) The biology and physiology of ageing. *The Western Journal of Medicine*. 153(6): 641–645.

telomerase levels can also help. But the quantum leaps in achieving longevity must come from methods that directly intervene in the ageing process. The use of stem cells and drugs like metformin and rapamycin show some promise, but biomedicine has some way to go yet to unlock the biological secrets of ageing.

From the TCM point of view, ageing results in the weakening of the five *zang* organs; the spleen has more difficulty in transforming food into nutrients and the body becomes more vulnerable to attack by external pathogens as defensive *qi* declines. There is greater tendency for emotional upsets and developing depression.

A weak *qi* constitution can succumb to infection that develops into heat excess syndrome, which is harder to treat with heat-clearing herbs as many of them may weaken *qi*. Ageing invariably increase blood stasis, especially if there has been prolonged chronic illness. There is also greater tendency for phlegm retention, which in turn can affect moods and stir up wind. There is also a greater tendency for an illness syndrome to transform into other syndromes. There is a general decline in healthy *qi* (*zheng qi*) and essence (*jing*) in the kidneys.

The Middle-Aged

These ageing processes accelerate in middle age. At this stage, the average person still looks good on the outside but in fact the internal organs, *qi* and blood are all heading south. As advanced age sets in, the body develops deficiency in *qi*, blood, and *yangqi*; essence and blood become increasingly depleted and spirits accordingly tend to be low; blood stasis and turbid phlegm worsen. Often the constitution of the elderly is deficient (asthenic) inside and appears excessive (sthenic) on the outside. After retirement, social status decline tends to demoralise the elderly; many become lonely, rejected and depressed or suffer from foul moods.

These inevitable consequences of ageing sound depressing and could give one little quarter for optimism. But there is a great deal that can be done following the principles of *yangsheng* to ameliorate these effects of ageing and, to some extent, slow them down.

For the middle-aged, it is important to start cultivating mind and spirit for tranquility. While seek material gains for a comfortable life after retirement get more urgent, doing so at the expense of a peaceful mind is likely to bring about a net negative result as work performance would be affected by a mind that is ill at ease with the state of the body and does not accept its unstoppable decline. Pursuit of fame and fortune should begin to play a less dominating role as one seeks fulfillment in social roles.

To avoid the onset of serious chronic illnesses, it is necessary to work moderately whilst creating more space for mental recreation and physical exercises like walking and biking, *taijiquan* and *qigong*.

Neijing's advice to keep regularity in living habits and avoiding overstrain takes on added urgency. Sexual excesses become less affordable as one's level of *yin* and *qi* and essence has already been partly depleted. The judicious use of tonics at this stage of life is needed to combat the ravages of the ageing process and avoid rapid decline into infirmity.

The Elderly

As we move into the elderly phase, it is important to attain a certain level of internal equanimity and come to terms with life and the inevitability of death. We seek peace of mind and adopt a positive outlook through activities that stimulate a passion for living. The company of good friends, appreciation of nature, and keeping the mind active through life-long learning all contribute to achieving greater longevity.

At this stage, diet and exercises must adapt to the reality of a weak spleen and stomach, hence it would be prudent to limit or avoid the consumption of cold or uncooked food. Eat warm cooked food that is easy to digest and choose medicated diet over medicine. Gentle exercises should aim to boost *qi* rather than muscular strength or cardiovascular performance. Competitive sports and exercising in bad weather would not be advisable for all but the extraordinarily fit elderly. There is now less space for late nights, and clothes and footwear must be appropriate to the weather at all times. Tonics should be taken, but only in smaller quantities and spread over longer periods.

10.4 Qigong and Taijiquan

Qigong (气功) is the practice of mental and physical skills that integrate body, breath and mind. Its practice involves both stretching of the muscles as well as concentration on breathing. *Qigong* involves meditation and breathing to promote the production and flow of blood and *qi* and strengthen the internal organs. 'Qi' in *qigong* refers to the *qi* of TCM, 'gong' means skill or technique, hence *qigong* was originally regarded as a method of building and moving *qi* in the body.

There are many forms of *qigong*. These include martial arts *qigong* which aims to strengthen body and master techniques for defense, Taoist *qigong* which cultivates mind and body to achieve the aim of prolonging life, and Confucian *qigong* which stresses the importance of fostering one's *qi* to cultivate the person, harmonise the family, and support governance of the state.

Medical *qigong* is the form of *qigong* that aims to prevent and treat disease, preserve health and prolong life. It historically evolved as a school in its own right from various forms of *qigong*. It comprises theory, manipulating skills, and clinical practice. It is guided by traditional Chinese philosophy, and incorporates ideas and methods from other schools and emphasises integration of dynamic and static exercise. Attention to the integration of three aspects of the exercise — movement, breathing and mind.

There are many schools of medical *qigong*. Among the popular ones are the Eight Brocades or *Baduanjing* (八段锦), comprising eight sets of graceful stretching exercises accompanied by breathing synchronised with its slow movements. Another school, derived largely from Taoist *qigong* is *Huichungong* (回春功) which literally means recovery of spring (youth). The movements are slow and deliberate and the practitioner appears in many of the movements to be performing a slow dance.

TCM believes that *qigong* can be used to prevent and assist in curing illnesses including the common cold, insomnia, digestive disorders, cardiovascular diseases, arthritis and sexual dysfunction. The rationale behind it is that it strengthens *qi* and promotes its smooth flow; at the same time the kidney function is improved with tonification of kidney essence and balancing of its *yin* and *yang*.

Taijiquan (太极拳)

Originally a form of martial art for offence as well as self-defense, many of its moves are lethal when executed fast. It was later adapted as a form of physical and mental training and health benefits. It uses the breathing and meditation techniques of *qigong*; thus it can also be understood as a martial art incorporating *qigong* techniques that has been transformed to slow graceful movements with tremendous health benefits akin to those derived from *qigong*. It combines movement with quiescence and is sometimes described as meditation by movement for its relaxing effects on the mind.

Taijiquan has the additional benefit over most *qigong* exercises of promoting physical balance, as movements are executed a great deal of time with only one foot on the floor. Hence it is encouraged as a gentle form of exercise that can help to prevent falls among the elderly.

10.5 Nutritional Principles of *Yangsheng*

There is a distinct difference between TCM dietary principles and those of Western nutritionists. The latter is based mainly on the classification of foods by carbohydrates, proteins, fats, fruits and vegetables. There has been considerable controversy of what constitutes the best diet in the West. There was a time when the 'food pyramid' recommended by the US Department of Agriculture advised people to eat carbohydrates as their main source of energy, avoid saturated fats and have good helpings of fruits and vegetables. More recently the thinking has changed towards avoiding minimising carbohydrates because they tend to be converted to harmful sugars, taking a moderate amount of saturated fats because only a very small amount of cholesterol in these fats are absorbed and turned into blood serum cholesterol. Eggs and dairy products including butter are back as healthy foods, and margarine (a trans fat) is to be avoided.

Types of Constitution

TCM advocates the principle that diet should be customised to the individual, as our nutritional needs vary according to our constitutions. TCM classifies people as belonging to one of nine kinds of constitution (Table 10.1).

Table 10.1   The nine kinds of constitution

1. Balanced and peaceful	平和体质
2. *Qi* deficiency	气虚体质
3. *Yang* deficiency	阳虚体质
4. Blood deficiency	血虚体质
5. *Yin* deficiency	阴虚体质
6. Phlegm-dampness	痰湿体质
7. Damp-heat	湿热体质
8. *Qi* stagnation	气郁体质
9. Blood stasis	血瘀体质

The first category, the balanced and peaceful constitution, represents the ideal healthy constitution. All the remaining eight constitutions have one or more syndromes that need to be corrected, and each person having one of these constitutions is deemed to be unwell. If the person has no clear clinical symptoms of disease, he is considered to be only sub-clinically ill (*yajiankang* 亚健康) as described in Chapter 2 of the book. People in these categories need to consume foods that help to correct their imbalances or improve flow within their bodies. Each other type of body constitution has its own set of defining symptoms.

Individuals who have a *qi* deficiency constitution is often characterised by weakness in the lung and spleen, and present symptoms such as a soft voice, fatigue, spontaneous sweating and poor appetite.

Blood deficiency constitutions comes with a pale complexion without lustre, pale lips, dizziness, heart palpitation or early thinning/dropping of hair.

The manifestations of *yang* deficiency constitutions are aversion to cold, frequent night urination and pale complexion whereas for the *yin* deficiency constitution are skinny, facial flush, dry mouth and throat, and vexation.

The symptoms of phlegm dampness and damp-heat body constitutions often have symptoms associated with the spleen and stomach because these organs are the source for the production of phlegm and dampness. Examples of symptoms for phlegm dampness constitution are a fat build, sluggishness, soft stools and sputum in the morning. For the damp heat constitution, the typical symptoms are aversion to heat, foul and sticky soft stools, a bloated stomach, and oily skin or scalp.

The symptoms for *qi* stagnation and blood stasis constitutions are commonly tightness or pain as flows are impeded. With the *qi* stagnation body constitution, a person is easily agitated or depressed and frequently experience chest tightness, whereas for blood stasis constitutions, the complexion is dark and dull and lips are dark.

The Role of Diet in Yangsheng

The role of diet in *yangsheng* may therefore be described as follows:

1. Restore normal body functions and remove deficiencies (扶正补虚). One should therefore use tonics according to deficiency in *qi*, blood, *yin* or *yang*.
2. Purge excess syndromes and eliminate pathogenic factors (泻实祛邪). Purge excess syndromes, which include stagnation of *qi*, blood stasis, and phlegm-dampness.
3. Prevent illness and promote longevity (防病益寿). By detecting syndromes early and resolving them with appropriate diet, one prevents disease from developing. This is known in TCM as *zhiweibing* (治未病), or healing the disease that has not yet occurred, and the ability of a physician

to achieve this in his patients is regarded as among the most treasured on his skills.

Other Yangsheng Dietary Principles

TCM *yangsheng* advises moderation in food and drink; eating about 80% full is believed to be better than having a full stomach at each meal. Eat meals at regular times; a hearty breakfast, a good lunch and a light dinner would be ideal.

When eating, concentrate on eating, chew the food well and try to eat while in a good mood. Taking a gentle stroll after meals helps the food go down and digest properly.

People with deficient spleen *yang* should eat warm cooked foods and avoid cold uncooked foods; with spleen deficiency and phlegm-dampness, avoid greasy fried foods; with asthma and skin allergies, avoid seafood and meat.

Combining Western and Chinese Wisdom in Diet

Western nutritionists rightly point out that one should avoid high glycemic-index carbohydrates and trans fats, moderate the amount of saturated fats, and higher consumption of vegetables especially those rich in fibre. The Mediterranean diet based on generous amounts of vegetables and nuts combined with moderate amounts of seafood and meat comes close to the present Western thinking on the ideal diet.

It is possible to combine this wisdom with that of Chinese *yangsheng* by following the above principles, at the same time choosing the particular foods in this diet that suit one's body constitution. For example a person with spleen *qi* weakness can still consume vegetables cooked rather than raw, and choose those vegetables that are not too cool or cold by

TCM classification. Likewise a person with blood deficiency could choose meats that have blood tonic effects and combine them with some herbs that are blood tonics.

In the next chapter we shall provide examples of foods that have the action of resolving various syndromes like heat, cold, dampness and deficiency of *qi*, blood, *yin* or *yang*. We then show you some appetizing recipes for cooked dishes, soups, herbal teas and porridges that will make food for *yangsheng* one of joys of living!

11

Medicated Foods and Teas

Healthy recipes that please the gourmet

The renowned Tang dynasty physician Sun Simiao 孙思邈 (581–682 AD) opined that the foundation of body health lay in food: "He who does not understand food is ill-suited to living." Since ancient times, the role of diet has been accorded prime importance in life cultivation; in particular, a diet that was not tailored to the individual person's constitution would be considered harmful to body health in the long run.

11.1 Characteristics of Medicated Food

Medicated food, commonly known as *yaoshan* (药膳), has herbs added to enhance its nutritional and health value, cooked in such a way as to be delicious and appetising in its own right. It is consistent with the fundamental principle that herbs and food come from the same source (*yaoshi tongyuan* 药食同源). The *Neijing* puts it this way: "If it is eaten on an empty stomach when one is well, it is considered as food; If it is eaten when one is unwell, it is regarded as a medicine" ("空腹食之为食物, 患者食之为药物").

TCM diet must take into account the particular syndromes that might be present at the time of enjoying medicated food, teas, and porridges. Many of the ingredients found in our daily meals are used as herbs by TCM physicians for therapeutic formulations.

The purpose of a medicated diet is to provide both nutritional and medicinal benefits in a meal. Less seasoning is usually used and most of the medicated diets are suitable for long-term consumption as their therapeutic actions are milder than those of medicinal decoctions as the dosage of medicinal herbs used is much less. To extract the nutrients from the foods as much as possible, medicated dishes are often prepared using cooking methods such as boiling, simmering, braising and steaming. These ways of cooking require the dish to be cooked over low heat for longer periods of time so as to ensure that the nutritious ingredients of the foods are captured in the meal. This explains why most medicated dishes come in the form of soups and porridges with all the goodness of the food ingredients locked in.

The medicated diet is both an art and a science. It involves culinary skills and many famous soups and cooked dishes have been modified and improved over time by specialists. The science of medicated diets draws on conventional Chinese medical principles. However, the medicinal properties of different foods have not been as well researched and documented as medical herbs, hence one should use the information in this chapter as a guide that has served the Chinese people well over many generations in their pursuit of health through *yangsheng*.

11.2 Food Ingredients

Nature and Flavour of Foods

As with herbs, foods have their own natures and flavours and generally one should try to have a balance of hot and cold foods. Food that is too hot damages *yin* fluids, and food that is too cold can harm *yangqi*, especially that of spleen and kidney. Examples of foods that are of hot/warm, cold/cool and neutral nature can be found in Table 11.1.

Table 11.1 List of foods with different properties

Hot/warm foods	Mutton, beef, chicken, pigeon, milk, carp, yellow croaker, snakeheaded fish (*yu sheng*), cuttle fish, sugar, peanut, sesame, soybean, rice, wheat, date, longan, lychee, mandarin orange, apple, onion garlic, chives, sweet potato, ginger, chilli, pepper
Cold/cool foods	Duck, honey, seaweed, kelp, mung bean, bitter gourd, lettuce, bamboo shoots, black fungus, banana, persimmon, pear, bean curd
Neutral foods	Pork, pork liver, chicken egg, jelly-fish skin, white fungus, water chestnut, red bean, pea, radish, lotus seed, lotus root, Chinese yam, spinach, carrot, tomato, Chinese cabbage, fresh kidney bean

Foods Classified by Their Actions

In order for the medicated food to be nutritious, it is important to adhere to the TCM principles. As with prescriptions, each of the ingredients has a role to play whether it is a monarch, minister, adjuvant or guiding role, and the choice of ingredients in the dish is dependent on the syndrome(s) that the dish is addressing. Besides taking into account of the therapeutic effects of the ingredients, the taste of the combination of herbs and food ingredients is a crucial factor for the selection of ingredients.

The therapeutic actions of foods can be classified into tonics to address deficiency syndromes and foods for removing pathogens to treat excess syndromes. The list of foods with medical benefits is extremely long. We provide below some examples of such foods and their corresponding actions in Tables 11.2 and 11.3.

We provide some examples below of three kinds of medicated food: porridges, soups and teas. Medicated food of course is available also in other forms such as fried, steamed or broiled dishes.

Table 11.2   List of tonic foods

Qi tonic foods	Rice, soybean, Chinese yam (*huaishan* 淮山), peanuts, *biantou* (扁豆) (hyacinth bean), millet, potato, carrot, date, quail and chicken eggs, pork tripe, beef, rabbit
Blood tonic foods	Pork liver, lamb, sea cucumber, raisins, red dates, blackstrap molasses, black fungus, spinach, carrot, *danggui*, dried longan
Yang tonic foods	Mutton, dog meat, sparrow, shrimp, walnut, Chinese chives (韭菜), sword bean (刀豆), black beans
Yin tonic foods	White fungus, mulberry fruit, bird's nest, pear, wolfberry seeds, turtle, black sesame (黑芝麻), most beans, especially millet (小米), duck, eggs, milk products

Table 11.3　List of foods for removing pathogens

Food for expelling exogenous pathogens	Ginger, shallot, fermented soybean
Food for clearing internal heat	Bittergourd, bitter vegetables, water melon, jue-cai (蕨菜), water chestnut
Food for clearing heat dampness	Eggplant, buckwheat (荞麦), purslane (马齿苋)
Food for warming the interior	Dry ginger, cinnamon, pepper, mutton, fennel (茴香)
Food for regulating *qi*	Sword bean, rose
Food for promoting blood flow and removing stasis	Hawthorn, wine, vinegar
Food for removing phlegm	Marine alga (海藻) kelp, laver (紫菜), sea tangle (海带), turnip, almond
Food for relieving cough	Almond, pear, gingko, loquat (枇杷), lily bulb
Food for alleviating anxiety	Lotus seeds, wheat, longan meat, lily bulb pig's heart
Food for promoting bowel movement	Almond, prune, seaweed, black sesame, banana, spinach, bamboo shoot
Food for relieving diarrhea	Dark plum, lotus seed

11.3 Porridges

"Porridge therapy" (*zhouliao* 粥疗) is used in *yangsheng* as well as for treatment of illnesses. Porridge has the special characteristic that rice after long boiling in watery form is easily digestible, hence is suitable for both healthy adults as well as children, the elderly and the sick. Rice, the main ingredient of porridge, is a mild *qi* tonic, and when porridge is served warm, it harmonises the stomach, tonifies the spleen, and clears the lung.

The two main kinds of rice used are *jingmi* (粳米) (round-grained non-glutinous rice) and *nuomi* (糯米) (polished glutinous rice). As mentioned in an ancient Chinese text, "*Jingmi* is the magic potion for nourishment and development, *nuomi* is ideal for warming and tonifying the stomach."[20] In the old days, most porridges use *jingmi*, although long-grained rice can sometimes be used as a substitute, and has similar therapeutic actions.

Below are three porridge recipes which incorporate the use of Chinese herbs for different therapeutic effects.

Nourishing Yin: Lily and Wolfberry Porridge (百合枸杞粥)

This porridge nourishes *yin* of the kidney, liver and lung, thereby resolving symptoms of *yin* deficiency, also clearing eyesight, improving production of fluids, and alleviating (dry) coughs.

Ingredients: Fresh lily bulb 30 g, wolfberry 30 g, round-grained rice 100 g, olive oil, and spring onions

Preparation Method:

1. Boil rice porridge for 1 hour.
2. Fry lily bulb in olive oil in deep pan.
3. Add boiled porridge and wolfberry to the pan, boil and simmer 30 minutes.
4. Add salt, pepper and spring onion to taste.

Strengthening the Spleen and Stomach: Chinese yam and Dangshen Porridge (山药党参粥)

This porridge helps to nourish the spleen and stomach by strengthening their functions, thereby alleviating poor digestion

---

[20] 《医药六书药性总义》:"粳米粥为资生化育神丹, 糯米粥为温养胃气妙品."

and dyspepsia. It can be an ideal daily breakfast for those who have weak spleen and stomach.

Ingredients: Fresh Chinese yam (山药) 30 g, cut into small chunks (less if dry), *dangshen* (党参) 10 g (sliced), *Jingmi* rice 60 g, a few slices of lean pork and egg white (optional)

Preparation Method:

1. Boil rice for 1 hour.
2. Add Chinese yam and *dangshen* and continue cooking for 1 hour.
3. Add sliced pork for a quick boil, then egg. Add salt and pepper to taste.

Tonifying Kidney Yang: Chestnut Porridge (栗子粥)

This porridge strengthens the kidney function by tonifying *yang*. Chestnut has the name of "fruit of kidney" (肾之果), hence it is suitable for those who have weak kidney constitution accompanied by aversion to cold and lower backaches. However, because of its warm nature, people with internal heat should avoid it.

Ingredients: Chestnut (10–15 g) (cut into small chunks), *jingmi* rice 100 g, wolfberry (10–20 g) (optional)

Preparation Method:

1. Boil rice for 30 minutes.
2. Add chestnut and continue cooking for 30 minutes to 1 hour until the chestnut is soft.
3. Add wolfberry seeds during the last 10 to 15 minutes. Serve warm. The addition of wolfberry seeds not only gives the porridge a sweet taste, but also provides a tonifying effect on the liver and kidney *yin*, thereby enhancing the action of strengthening the kidney functions.

11.4 Soup Recipes

Soups are generally regarded as nutritious foods because all the nutrients are infused in it after boiling and simmering for hours. As such, it is always good to drink soup slowly and before meals so as to allow efficient absorption of nutrients, especially for the case of medicated diets which have medicinal effects as well. We will be showing some simple recipes for different body constitutions, which you can try out at home. These recipes are just a guide on the types of ingredients to use for the various types of body constitutions or syndromes. You may find it interesting to modify the recipes to make them more appealing to your taste!

Clearing Heat and Dampness: Job's Tears and Green Bean Soup (苡仁绿豆汤)

Ingredients: Job's tears (*yiyiren* 薏苡仁) 100 g, green beans (绿豆) 50 g, dried tangerine peel (*chenpi* 陈皮) 5–10 g

Preparation Method:

1. Soak Job's tears and green beans in water for at least an hour.
2. After soaking, put them and dried tangerine peel in a pot and add water (about 1500 ml).
3. Cook until Job's tears and green beans turn soft. If preferred, you may add some rock sugar for a sweeter taste. Serve warm.

This soup is suitable for those who have a heat-dampness body constitution (湿热体质). It helps to expel toxins, clear summer-heat and resolve dampness. The dosage of Job's tears (monarch) is the highest as its action of clearing heat-dampness is the strongest. Dried tangerine peel is used sparingly because of its bitter taste; it acts as an adjuvant role by promoting the flow of *qi* which is often impeded by dampness. The addition of dried tangerine peel also helps to protect the spleen and stomach from the cool nature of Job's tears and green beans, which enhances the action in clearing summer-heat. A person who has a weak spleen and stomach should avoid drinking this soup. For those who prefer the dish to be more filling, we can add more Job's tears or green beans to make it more like porridge.

Resolving Dampness and Phlegm: Gordon Fruit, Lotus Seed and Job's Tears Soup (芡实莲子苡仁汤)

Ingredients: Pork ribs 300 g (chopped into small chunks), lotus seeds (莲子) 20 g, gordon fruit (*qianshi* 芡实) 30 g, Job's tears 30 g, dried tangerine peel (陈皮) 5 g, 1 ginger

Preparation Method:

1. Soak lotus seeds, gordon fruit, Job's tears and dried tangerine peel in water.
2. After soaking, put the pork and herbs in a claypot.
3. Add water and ginger. Bring to boil.
4. Continue to simmer for 2 hours. Add salt to taste. Serve warm.

This soup mainly helps to resolve dampness and phlegm, thereby suitable for those who have a phlegm-dampness body constitution (痰湿体质). Gordon fruit has the action of removing dampness and lotus seeds help to tonify the spleen so that it will prevent the production of phlegm and dampness. As compared to the above soup, this soup is not as cooling and has a harmonising effect on the spleen and stomach functions because of the presence of lotus seeds, gordon fruit and dried tangerine peel. Generally, this soup can be used in most individuals because the therapeutic actions are milder and the coolness of Job's tears is mitigated by the warm nature of the ginger and dried tangerine peel. Pork ribs are added to enhance the taste of the soup. As *qianshi* has an arresting (holding back) action, people who have constipation should avoid eating this dish.

Promoting Blood Flow: Chinese Angelica, Tianqi and Black Chicken Soup (当归田七乌鸡汤)

Ingredients: 1 black chicken, Chinese angelica (*danggui* 当归) 15 g, *Sanqi* (三七) 5g, 1 ginger (optional)

Preparation Method:

1. Soak *sanqi* and *danggui*.
2. Put black chicken and the rest of the ingredients into a pot.
3. Add salt and just enough water to cover the black chicken.
4. Steam over high heat for 3 hours.

This soup helps to promote blood flow, remove stasis and nourish blood and is suitable for those who have a blood stasis body constitution (瘀血体质). Black chicken is a tonic food for *qi* and blood; *danggui* nourishes blood and *sanqi* promotes blood flow and removes stasis without damaging the *qi* in the body. This soup is warm and not suitable for those who have the heat syndrome. Ginger can be removed if this soup is too hot for your liking. Individuals who have *yin* deficiency and weak stomachs should avoid taking this soup.

Black Chicken Soup for Nourishing Blood (养血乌鸡汤)

Ingredients: Black chicken (乌鸡), Chinese angelica (*danggui* 当归) 10 g, astragalus (*huangqi* 黄芪) 20 g, *chuanxiong* (川芎) 6 g, *shengdihuang* (生地黄) 10 g, red dates (*dazao* 大枣) 10 g

Preparation Method:

1. Soak all the herbs in 2000 ml of water.
2. Blanch the black chicken and put into the pot of water.
3. Bring it to boil and continue to cook it over low heat for another 45–60 minutes.
4. Add salt to taste. Serve warm

This dish is suitable for individuals who have a blood deficiency constitution (血虚体质). It mainly nourishes blood and also has a mild action in promoting blood flow with the addition of *chuanxiong*. Although *huangqi* is a *qi* tonic, it is added to assist in the production of blood, since *qi* is required to produce blood. *Shengdihuang* with its cool nature, is added to mitigate the warming nature of the soup, and has a mild action in nourishing *yin*. Compared to *bazhentang* (八珍汤), this soup is not as warm in nature and can also be used for women who have just finished menstruation to help replenish blood. Individuals who have heat syndrome should avoid drinking this soup.

Soup for Nourishing Yin (沙参玉竹鸭肉汤)

Ingredients: Duck 600 g (cut into big pieces), *beishashen* (北沙参) 50 g, *yuzhu* (玉竹) 50 g, ginger 2 pieces

Preparation Method:

1. Soak both *beishashen* and *yuzhu* in 2000 ml of water for 30 minutes.
2. Add the duck and bring to a boil.
3. Lower the heat, skim fat from the surface of the soup and continue to simmer for about 30 minutes. Serve warm.

This soup nourishes *yin*, especially lung and stomach *yin* and is good for those who have a *yin* deficiency body constitution (阴虚体质). Duck has the action of nourishing *yin* and *beishashen* and *yuzhu* are both *yin* tonics, which also help to promote the production of fluids. This soup is good for prevention of dry throat and cough, especially during autumn in temperate countries, as it helps to nourish and moisten the lung. With the addition of ginger which helps to warm the spleen and stomach, this soup will not be as cooling and it can be consumed by most people.

Black Bean Soup for Tonifying Kidney (黑豆干貝山药湯)

Ingredients: *Duzhong* (杜仲) 10 g, black beans 50 g (soak for 1 hour), fresh Chinese yam (*shanyao* 山药) 200–250 g (skin removed, cut into cubes), red dates (*dazao* 大枣) 50 g, scallop 30–50 g, rice wine 30 ml.

Preparation Method:

1. Add black beans and scallop into 1500 ml of water.
2. Boil over low heat for 1 hour.
3. Add red dates and Chinese yam. Cook for another 5 minutes.
4. Add rice wine and salt to taste. Serve warm.

The main therapeutic action of this soup is to tonify kidney *yang*, hence it is suitable for *yang* deficiency body constitution (阳虚体质). Both *duzhong* and black beans have the actions of tonifying *yang* and strengthening the kidney; Chinese yam nourishes the spleen and kidney, thereby this soup takes care two of the more important *zang* organs in Chinese medicine: the prenatal (kidney) and postnatal (spleen) base of life. Strengthening the kidney helps to prevent premature greying of hair and hair loss.

Strengthening Qi: Chicken Soup for Qi (参芪鸡汤)

Ingredients: Chicken 200 g, *dangshen* (党参) 15 g, astragalus (*huangqi* 黄芪) 10 g, fresh Chinese yam (*shanyao* 山药) 100–150 g (skin removed, cut into cubes)

Preparation Method:

1. Soak the herbs in 1500 ml of water for 30 minutes.
2. Add the blanched chicken and bring it to boil.
3. Add the fresh Chinese yam and continue to simmer over low heat for 30 to 50 minutes.
4. Add salt to taste. Serve warm.

Chicken is known to be a food for improving *qi*, which explains why this soup is for *qi* deficiency body constitution (气虚体质). In addition, the soup also comprises *qi* tonics such as *dangshen*, *huangqi* and Chinese yam to enhance the therapeutic effect of replenish *qi*, especially that of spleen and lung since spleen is the source of *qi* production and lung governs *qi*. This soup is good for those who always feel weak and is a dish which can be cooked for the family once in a while to replenish body *qi*.

11.5 Herbal Teas

Similar to medicated diet, herbal teas are also customised to the body's condition. The herbs used are mostly of plant origin as they generally taste better and are easier for the extraction of the desired ingredients. Depending on the plant parts, certain herbal teas can easily be made by steeping them in hot water whereas others may need boiling. Herbs that are flowers, leaves or fleshy fruits can be used for steeping whereas roots, barks, stems and seeds often require some boiling. Unless it is required by your body condition, it is not advisable to drink the same herbal tea on a daily basis. It should be taken in moderation and stopped when one feels better, especially for cooling herbal teas as they may harm the spleen and stomach in the long run. An exception can be made for teas that are neutral in nature and have tonifying effects. These can be taken more regularly such as two to three times a week.

Below are a few tantalizing herbal teas recipes for your enjoyment. These quantities of herbs used are for one teapot serving.

Clear Vision Tea (清热明目茶)

Herbs: Chrysanthemum flower 8 g, mulberry leaves 3–6 g, wolfberry seeds 3–6 g

Preparation Method: Steep the herbs in hot water

With the actions of clearing liver fire to improve vision, this tea is ideal for those who stay up late at night and suffer from dry and reddened eyes due to liver fire. Chrysanthemum flowers and mulberry leaves help to clear the liver fire while wolfberry seeds help to nourish liver *yin*. Some red dates can be added to give the tea a natural sweet taste. As this tea is cooling, it is advisable not to take it for too long.

Nourishing and Calming Tea (养血宁心茶)

Herbs: Longan meat 6 g, lily bulb 5 g, red dates 3 pieces, wolfberry seeds 3–6 g

Preparation Method: Steep the herbs in hot water or boil the herbs for a stronger concentration.

Having difficulty falling asleep and feeling vexed these days? This tea may be able to solve your sleeping problem if the underlying syndrome is heart blood and *yin* deficiency. Longan meat and red dates nourish blood to calm the heart and mind for a sounder sleep; and lily bulb, which has a cool nature, can help to put out the deficiency fire resulted from the weakened *yin*.

Longevity Tea (寿比南山茶)

Ingredients: *Huangqi* (黄芪) 4-6 g, *huangjing* (黄精) 6 g, *zhigancao* (炙甘草) 3-5 g, wolfberry seeds 3-6 g

Preparation Method: After boiling, cook for 30 to 40 minutes. Wolfberry seeds can be added in the last 15 minutes.

The two precious ingredients in this tea, *huangqi* and *huangjing* help to enhance vital energy and longevity by tonifying *qi* and essence. *Huangjing* nourishes lung, spleen and kidney which can help to retard the ageing process. As pointed out in an earlier chapter, research has suggested that *huangqi* can help to slow down ageing by boosting the body enzyme telomerase. *Zhigancao* is a mild *qi* tonic to further enhance the *qi* tonifying action. As *huangqi* and *huangjing* are roots, it is recommended to boil them for a stronger effect. Wolfberry is added in the last 15 minutes as it will have a sour taste if it is cooked for too long.

Digestion Tea (消食降脂茶)

Ingredients: Hawthorn 6 g, *danshen* (丹参) 4-6 g, *zhigancao* 3-5 g, rock sugar (optional)

Preparation Method: After boiling, cook for 15-20 minutes.

This tea assists in digesting a rich and heavy meal. It can be easily made by boiling three herbs with hawthorn berry as the main ingredient for promoting digestion of fats/lipids. *Danshen* plays a ministerial role by promoting blood flow and removing stasis. As hawthorn berry is sour, individuals who have weak stomach should avoid this tea before meals. Pregnant ladies should also drink this tea with caution as hawthorn has the action of promoting blood flow. With its sweet flavour, *zhigancao* is added to mitigate the sourness of the tea. This tea can also be used in individuals who have mild coronary heart disease as clinical research suggests that both *danshen* and hawthorn may help to slow down atherosclerosis.

Yin Nourishing and Thirst Quenching Tea (养阴止渴茶)

Ingredients: *Dendrobium* (*shihu* 石斛) 6 g, *yuzhu* (玉竹) 3 g, American ginseng 4–5 pieces, wolfberry 3–6 g

Preparation Method: Steep the herbs in hot water or boil the herbs for a stronger concentration.

This tea mainly contains *yin* tonics that help to promote the production of body fluids. It quenches thirst due to *yin* deficiency, which results in deficiency fire, thereby leading to thirst and dryness in the throat and mouth. Dendrobium and *yuzhu* help to nourish stomach and kidney *yin* and replenish fluids in the body. American ginseng not only nourishes *yin* but also tonifying *qi*, hence this tea also has a *qi* tonifying action.

Complexion Enhancing Tea (贵妃养颜茶)

Ingredients: Rose flowers 4 g, jasmine flower 2 g, red dates 3–4 pieces

Preparation Method: Steep the herbs in hot water

A popular tea among the ladies, this fragrant flora tea helps to enhance one's complexion by promoting better *qi* and blood flow. With good flows in the body, there is sufficient blood to nourish and moisten the skin, bringing a healthy pink glow to the skin.

12

Nip It in the Bud

The prevention and management of chronic diseases

To illustrate how TCM methods are applied to some common chronic illnesses, we examine briefly its use in coronary heart disease, stroke, diabetes, digestive disorders, depression and cancer. These conditions have been chosen because TCM treatment in each case provides an interesting complement or alternative to Western medicine. TCM physicians regularly encounter patients who may not have found satisfactory results with Western medicine for such ailments and seek alternative treatments. The objective here is to show how TCM methods have been used in a wide variety of clinical work and offer a comparison with biomedical methods.

12.1 Coronary Heart Disease

In most instances coronary heart disease involves the narrowing of blood vessels supplying nutrients and oxygen to the heart. This narrowing is caused by dietary, genetic, ageing and lifestyle factors with build-up of fatty plaque on arterial walls. Angina pain can occur when blood supply is inadequate and cardiac arrest when there is constriction or blockage.

TCM interprets coronary heart disease as an impediment to or blockage of the free flow of *qi* and blood. The condition is classified under 'chest blockage with heart pain' (*xiongbi xintong* 胸痹心痛) in TCM textbooks and attributed to one or more of seven underlying syndromes, of which the most common are deficiency of heart *qi* and blood stasis.

The syndrome deficiency of heart *qi* is identified by symptoms of dull pain in the chest, heart palpitations, shortness of breath which worsens upon exertion, fatigue and sweating without exertion; the tongue is pale and slightly swollen, with tooth indentations and thin white fur; the pulse is slow, weak and thready or slow and irregular. The syndrome of 'blood stasis' has symptoms of stabbing pain or angina pain in the chest, sometimes spreading to the back and shoulders; it can be accompanied by prolonged 'chest oppression'; the tongue is dark with ecchymosis (bluish-black marks) and thin fur; pulse is wiry and astringent, or rapid and intermittent/irregular.

In the absence of other syndromes associated with heart disease, the first syndrome of deficient heart *qi* is consistent with early or mild coronary heart disease. Blood stasis syndrome is usually found in more advanced stages of the disease when significant atherosclerosis has set in. Deficiency of heart *qi* usually occurs in the early stages, and the additional syndrome of blood stasis sets in as the disease progresses, hence we can regard *qi* deficiency as the root syndrome and blood stasis as the consequent syndrome of disease progression.

Accordingly, TCM treatment for the first syndrome consists of strengthening the body's *qi* level and promoting (regulating) its flow through *qigong* and *taiji* exercises, as well as diets containing foods and herbs that tonify *qi*, such as American ginseng, Chinese yam (*huaishan*), Astragalus (*huangqi*), *ginseng, dangshen and sanqi*. A typical prescription formulation, appropriately modified to suit each patient's condition, would be *Baoyuan Tang* (保元汤) combined with *Ganmaidazao Tang* (甘麦大枣汤). The first uses ginseng and Astragalus as the main components for boosting *qi* levels. The latter uses *xiaomai* (小麦) or wheat as the monarch herb to nourish heart *yin* and roasted liquorice (*zhigancao*) as the minister herb to promote flow along the heart meridian, invigorating the heart and tranquilising the mind. For the second syndrome, TCM treatment would typically encourage the consumption of foods and herbs that improve blood circulation and reduce blood stasis. These would include *danshen* (丹参), hawthorn berries (*shanzha*), red yeast rice (*hongqumi* 红曲米), *chuanxiong* (川芎), *safflower* (*honghua*), peach kernel (*taoren* 桃仁), black fungus vegetable, turmeric and pomegranate fruit.[21] In biomedical terms, these herbs are known to have mild vasodilating effects, rendering transient improved blood flow and symptomatic relief from angina pains. In the TCM framework, such vasodilating effects are only symptoms of more lasting changes brought about by 'resolving

---

[21] Noted advocate of natural healing, Andrew Weil MD recommends the regular consumption of black fungus for coronary heart health. See Weil (1995:166).

blood stasis', a claim which implies slower build-up of plaque and less impediment to blood flow. A typical prescription for blood stasis syndrome in the chest is the 'Decoction for Removing Blood Stasis in the Chest' (*Xuefu Zhuyu Tang* 血府逐瘀汤). This formulation contains 11 herbs, with *honghua* and *taoren* as monarch drugs, and *chuanxiong* as one of the minister drugs.

In recent years the classical Chinese formulation '*Danshen* Dripping Pills' (*Fufang Danshen Diwan* 复方丹参滴丸) for alleviating blood stasis and improving blood flow has completed Phase 2 FDA trials and is awaiting final approval for use in the treatment of coronary heart disease. This formulation contains *danshen*, *sanqi* and *bingpian* (冰片). A combination of blood stasis and *qi* deficiency has been used to explain restenosis of coronary arteries after patients received stents in their coronary arteries. Some success has been claimed for preventing restenosis by putting such patients on formulations promoting *qi* and resolving blood stasis. It combines tonification for heart *qi* using ginseng and astragalus, reducing blood stasis with *chuanxiong*, safflower, and *taoren*, and alleviating blockages using *gualou* (瓜蒌).

Compared to Western treatments using the nitrates for vasodilation, blood thinners (like aspirin) to reduce the risk of blood clots, and surgical interventions like angioplasty and bypass surgery, TCM treatments are slower and cannot deal effectively with acute angina or emergency situations of coronary infarction. But they could be useful either as complementary treatment or as an alternative to surgical intervention. TCM treatments, with proper medical advice recognising drug contraindications and the condition of the patient, can and are being administered alongside Western treatments. TCM approaches of management of heart conditions using medicated diets and Chinese exercises can complement Western methods such as maintaining low cholesterol levels, exercises for cardiovascular fitness, and a diet rich in fibre and low in saturated and trans fats and rich in fresh fruits and vegetables to promote endothelial health. The use of Chinese herbal supplements to improve *qi* and reduce blood stasis may be of significant help in reducing arterial wall inflammation hence make an important contribution to the prevention and treatment of coronary heart disease.

12.2 Hypertension and Stroke

With ageing, atherosclerosis sets in as arteries narrow with plaque on their walls. The likelihood of suffering a stroke rises almost exponentially after the age of 65. Both Western medicine and TCM treat patients to prevent strokes and, if a stroke has occurred, to ameliorate its effects and improve quality of life. The approaches taken by the two systems of medicine appear radically different, but in fact have underlying commonalities.

Of the two major kinds of strokes, the ischaemic stroke and the haemorrhagic stroke, the former is by far the more common, being precipitated by sudden impeded blood flow in an artery of the brain. This could be caused by clotting at the artery (thrombosis), or a detached clot from another location — usually the heart or the carotid artery — that lodges itself within the artery (embolism), cutting off oxygen supply to part of the brain. A haemorrhagic stroke results from rupture of an artery wall, leading to cerebral haemorrhage, and it is commonly correlated with degenerative disease of the arteries and hypertension. The use of blood thinners like warfarin can also raise the risk of a haemorrhagic stroke.

Western medicine attributes strokes to a combination of risk factors, which may include hypertension, smoking, excessive cholesterol (LDL) levels, and diabetes. Heart arrhythmia in the form of atrial fibrillation can also produce clots that travel to the brain.

TCM views that the underlying conditions predisposing a person to strokes involve the endogenous wind (*feng* 风) pathogen; hence the Chinese term for stroke is *zhong feng* (中风), or 'attack by wind'. Endogenous wind may arise from one or more of several factors, which include (a) weakness of *yin* and blood giving rise to liver heat and wind; (b) overwork and strain stirring up liver wind; (c) inappropriate diet that creates warm phlegm in the spleen, generating endogenous wind; (d) emotional stress particularly anger triggering fire and the production of harmful wind.

One or more of a number of TCM syndrome combinations may be observed with strokes, depending on the nature of the stroke and the stage of progression, whether at the onset, in the immediate aftermath, or during the longer term debilitated phase of the patient. At the onset and immediate aftermath stage, hyperactivity of liver *yang*, phlegm with wind, and stirring of liver wind (*ganfeng neidong* 肝风内动) are the common syndromes. At the later recovery stages, phlegm and blood stasis are often present, and the patient may suffer from severe *qi* deficiency and weakness of the liver and kidney.

Tianma Gouteng Yin (天麻钩藤饮) with suitable variations to suit the patient is most often used in the early stages whilst tonics with ingredients added for resolving blood stasis such as *Buyang Huanwu Tang* (补阳还五汤) are administered in the recovery stages. Thus, treatment of these TCM syndromes associated with strokes follows the principle of customising therapy to the syndrome and the constitution of the patient. Treatment usually combines herbal prescriptions, acupuncture and *tuina*, and is continually varied as the internal state of the patient changes and new syndromes are exhibited.

TCM theory explains that acupuncture helps the rehabilitation process by enhancing flow of *qi* and blood in the body, leading to better recovery of motor skills and overall physical functioning by inducing beneficial changes in the blood flow to the brain. Common points used in post-stroke acupuncture treatment include *taichong* (太冲), *hegu* (合谷), *renzhong* (人中), *baihui* (百会), *sanyinjiao* (三阴交), *neiguan* (内关), *yanglingquan* (阳陵泉) and *quchi* (曲池). These acupoints can also be used in the treatment of hypertension.

Exercises like *qigong* and *taijiquan*, for patients with sufficient mobility, are believed to enhance recovery from post-stroke disabilities. Social interaction within *qigong* groups may also help to improve patient morale and nurture the positive emotions that facilitate recovery.

Western treatments for stroke rely heavily on blood coagulants like warfarin to prevent recurrence and on physiotherapy for rehabilitation. Chinese treatments directly address the prevailing syndromes at each stage of the evolution of the illness. In the early aftermath of a stroke, there is an emphasis on calming endogenous wind, in the later stages, the focus is on resolving phlegm and blood stasis, while in the rehabilitation and recovery phase, this shifts to tonics for *qi*, blood and the *yin* of the liver and kidney. Chinese exercises work on improving blood and *qi* circulation, postural robustness and joint mobility, less on building muscular strength. It would appear that a combination of Western and Chinese treatments can secure better results for the patient than a strict adherence to one regimen. When treatments are combined, there must be appropriate cognisance of drug compatibility. For example, some Chinese herbs have mild anticoagulant properties that may excessively enhance the effect of Western anticoagulant drugs.

12.3 Diabetes Mellitus

Diabetes Mellitus is a disorder of carbohydrate metabolism in which sugars in the body are not oxidised to produce energy due to lack of insulin leading to high blood glucose (sugar) level. It is one of the fastest-growing diseases in developed countries, some of which are witnessing epidemic-like growth.

There are two types of diabetes: Type 1 diabetes is an autoimmune disease in which the body's own immune system attacks the pancreas, thereby leading a decrease in insulin production whereas type 2 diabetes is a lifestyle disease which is attributed to poor dietary habits and an inactive lifestyle, with obesity as one of the major risk factors.

In type 2 diabetes, the body develops insulin resistance to glucose and is consequently unable to carry glucose into the body's cells either for storage or metabolism. In the longer run, insulin production drops and type 2 diabetes is developed. The exact cause for type 2 diabetes is still yet to be found even though recent research has suggested that chronic inflammation could be the one. The usual signs and symptoms for both types of diabetes are thirst, hunger, weight loss, frequent urination, and lethargy although there are some diabetic people who do not show any symptoms.

There is no exact equivalent of diabetes in TCM. The symptoms associated with diabetes resemble closely a condition recorded in the *Neijing* and in modern TCM texts as *xiaoke* (消渴); *xiao* (消) means exhausting of the body's nutrients and *ke* (渴) means thirst. This term captures the classic symptoms of *xiaoke* as excessive thirst, frequent urination, hunger pangs, weight loss and sugar in the urine; these are similar to the typical symptoms of diabetes. It is possible however for a patient to have the symptoms of *xiaoke* but blood tests do not show an abnormal sugar level; or to have high sugar level and not exhibit *xiaoke* symptoms. In modern TCM usage which has been influenced by biomedical terminology, the term *tangniaobing* (糖尿病) is commonly used to refer to diabetes and is not strictly differentiated from *xiaoke*. TCM attributes *xiaoke* symptoms to *yin* deficiency, which is accompanied by 'asthenic fire' and dryness (阴虚燥热). The illness can be categorised by dysfunctions of a particular organ and the TCM syndrome associated with it. All categories of the illness have in common symptoms of thirst, hunger and frequent urination to different degrees. The *zang* organ which is affected in the early stage of *xiaoke* is the lung which has the underlying syndrome of lung heat with dryness (肺热津伤), also known as the upper trunk *xiaoke* (上消). The main symptom is thirst even after drinking, accompanied by excessive and frequent urination, dry tongue and mouth, vexatiousness, thin yellowish fur on the tongue with strong and fast pulse.

As the illness progresses, it affects the stomach and results in middle trunk *xiaoke* (中消) which can have two possible syndromes: (i) Exuberance of stomach fire (胃热炽盛) which is characterised by hunger pangs, abnormally thin or weak, constipation with dry stools and yellowish fur; (ii) Deficiency in spleen *qi* and *yin* (气阴亏虚) which usually manifests into intense thirst, abnormally huge appetite with loose stools, skinny, fatigue, light-red tongue with dry white fur and weak pulse. The late stage of *xiaoke* usually damages the kidney and results in lower trunk *xiaoke* (下消), with the syndrome of kidney *yin* deficiency (肾阴亏虚). The main symptoms are excessive and frequent urination, cloudy urine, dry lips, skinny, weak knees, soreness in the lower back, dry itchy skin, red tongue with little or no fur and a thready rapid pulse.

The general TCM treatment approach is to resolve the syndromes that are presented rather than the disease directly. This may require replenishing *yin*, moisturising dryness and removing the heat with the use of *yin* tonics.

In upper trunk *xiaoke*, the formulation used is modified *xiaoke fang* (消渴方) which comprises mainly *tianhuafen* (天花粉), *maidong* (麦冬) and *shengdi* (生地) to nourish *yin* and promote the production of fluids to quench thirst; *zhimu* (知母) and *huangqin* (黄芩) to purge fire. For middle trunk *xiaoke*, the typical formulation to address the exuberance of stomach fire syndrome is *yunujian* (玉女煎) which has *shudihuang* (熟地黄) and *maidong* to nourish *yin,* and *zhimu* and *shigao* (石膏) to purge stomach fire; the formulation for deficiency in spleen *qi* and *yin* is modified *qiweibaizhusan* (七味白术散) which comprises mainly spleen *qi* tonics such as *dangshen* (党参), *baizhu* (白术) and *zhigancao* (炙甘草), and *yin* tonics such as *maidong* and *tianmendong* (天门冬). For lower trunk *xiaoke*, the formulation to treat kidney *yin* deficiency would be the classical *liuweidihuangtang* (六味地黄汤). You will recall from Chapter 8 that this formulation contains the three tonics (*shudihuang and shanzhuyu* (山茱萸), both of which nourish kidney *yin*, and *shanyao* (山药), which nourishes both the kidney and spleen and three purgatives to douse deficiency fire and drain dampness (*mudanpi* 牡丹皮, *zexie* 泽泻 and *fuling* 茯苓).

Blood stasis syndrome may be seen in late stage diabetic patients with complications such as nephropathy, retinopathy, and chronic heart disease. In the course of TCM treatment, herbs with blood promoting and removing stasis actions are therefore added to the formulation accordingly.

Besides the above formulations, research has suggested that there are some herbs in TCM that may be helpful in the control and management of blood glucose level. These include *huangqi* (黄芪), purslane (*machixian* 马齿苋), *shanzhuyu* and cinnamon bark (*rougui* 肉桂). As a holistic system that places strong emphasis on achieving a balanced lifestyle, diet and emotions as the basis of good health, TCM can play an effective role in the prevention and management of diabetes.

12.4 Digestive Disorders and the Irritable Bowel Syndrome

Li Dongyuan (李东垣) of the Jin-Yuan dynasties focused on care of the digestive system for health and longevity, and damage to the spleen and stomach is the root cause of most illnesses. The TCM spleen governs the processing and transforming food into nutrients that feed other organs and the rest of the body, pairing with the stomach in its work. The spleen nourishes the body and replenishes the store of *qi*, blood and essence or *jing* in the vital organs. Growth and development in TCM theory are governed mainly by the kidney. By providing nutrients to the kidney to replenish the store of *qi* and *jing*, the spleen serves as the foundation of postnatal health.

In TCM theory, spleen functions are inhibited by dampness, which is characterised by 'stickiness' that impedes the flow of *qi*, resulting in *qi* stagnation in the abdomen. With weak *qi* and/or *qi* stagnation, dampness accumulates further, food is not properly digested, and there could be resultant generation and accumulation of phlegm. Improper diet such as oily and fried foods and brooding accompanied by anxiety are the leading factors that damage the spleen, resulting in gastrointestinal disorders such as poor appetite, a bloated abdomen, wind, loose stools, and the discomforts of the irritable bowel syndrome. The high incidence of digestive disorders in high-stress societies like New York, Beijing and Singapore may well be associated with stressful lifestyles that harm the spleen.

Herbal supplements used to strengthen spleen functions include dried tangerine peels (*chenpi*), *sharen* and *banxia* which are thought to smoothen the flow of spleen *qi* and resolve dampness and phlegm; *dangshen*, wild yam (*shanyao*), *huangqi* and red dates are used to tonify spleen *qi*. These herbs can be used as food ingredients for spleen-healthy meals, although *sharen* and *banxia* are not so tasty and tend to be used more in medical prescriptions. A delicious nourishing rice porridge with *huangqi*, red dates and wild yam can be used to maintain healthy functioning of the spleen and stomach.

Common formulations for spleen disorders include *Sijunzi Tang*, *Shenling Baizhu San*, and *Xiangsha Liujunzi Tang*.[22] These formulations combine *qi* tonics with *qi* regulation and removal of dampness.

Irritable Bowel Syndrome

The Irritable Bowel Syndrome (IBS) is a recurrent condition with abdominal pains and constipation and/or diarrhoea, often with bloating of the abdomen and dyspepsia. There is no detectable structural disease. It can continue for years. The condition is often associated with stress or anxiety and may follow an episode of intestinal infection. From the point of view of Western medicine, 'the cause is unknown'.[23]

TCM regards IBS (*changyiji zonghezheng* 肠易激综合征) as a condition associated with imbalances and/or stagnation in the spleen. It is not a disease in its own right, but one of several manifestations of imbalance and *qi* stagnation in the spleen. This could take the form of dampness in the spleen when spleen *qi* is weak or does not flow properly, the result of improper diet or exposure to the dampness pathogen. It can also be the consequence of an 'exuberant' liver over-restraining the spleen, a possible condition explained by the five-element model, causing the spleen to malfunction in its digestive role. The exuberant liver is often the result of stress and anxiety, causing stagnation in liver *qi* flow and progressing to 'liver fire'.

---

[22] See Annex 2 for these formulations.
[23] Oxford Concise Medical Dictionary (2007:380).

IBS is frequently encountered in TCM practice especially among city dwellers in high-stress environments. Stress harms the liver, stoking exuberance and fire. Excessive consumption of fried and high-fat foods that are difficult to digest make a veritable breeding ground for spleen dampness.

TCM treatment for IBS comprises mainly resolving spleen dampness with herbs and formulations like *Xiangsha Liujunzi Tang*, or calming the liver with *Xiaoyaosan* with variations customised to the condition of the patient.[24] IBS-like conditions are frequently encountered in TCM clinical work and there is considerable anecdotal evidence of the efficacy of TCM treatments. Some recent clinical trials have claimed success with such treatments.

12.5 Depression

Depression in Western medicine is a mood disorder "characterised by the pervasive and persistent presence of core and somatic symptoms on most days for at least two weeks."[25] Core symptoms include impairment of motivation, energy, enjoyment and memory, insomnia, loss of appetite and libido, and mood swings. A definitive diagnosis of clinical depression is difficult because symptoms vary greatly across individuals. Western medicine views genetics, chronic illnesses and stress as possible underlying causes of depression. Depressive states may be accompanied by low levels of neurotransmitters in the para-sympathetic nervous system. Treatment would involve use of anti-depressants, cognitive behavioural therapy and/or psychotherapy.

---

[24] See Annex 2 for these formulations.
[25] Oxford Concise Medical Dictionary (2007:195).

TCM does not have an exact equivalent of depression as an illness. The word *yu* (郁) means stagnation or the absence of smooth flow of *qi* in the body and the TCM term *yubing* (郁病) refers to a group of conditions arising from blocked flows of *qi* and/or blood in the body, leading to a variety of symptoms ranging from sadness and anxiety to vile tempers and autism. *Yubing* does not therefore correspond exactly to the Western medical meaning of depression and is best viewed as a class of syndromes, many of them exhibiting the symptoms associated with depression in biomedicine.

A common cause of *qi* stagnation in TCM theory is the emotional factor. Excessive anger and emotional stress leads to stagnation of liver *qi*, which may progress into liver fire. Anxiety may result in the stagnation of spleen *qi*, which in turn may encourage production of dampness and phlegm that further impede the flow of *qi*. Among menopausal and post-partum women who tend to be low in *yin* and *qi*, weakness or deficiency of blood and nourishment to the heart are commonly encountered. *Yubing* symptoms include frequent abrupt mood swings, paranoia, anxiety and panic attacks.

The TCM approach to treatment of *yubing* involves identifying the blockages and imbalances and resolving them with herbal medications and/or acupuncture to restore *qi* flow. For mild cases, herbs with soothing and calming effects, targeting the particular syndrome exhibited by the patient, may be helpful. Herbs that help to improve *qi* flows include *chaihu* (柴胡), *xiangfu* (香附), *foshou* (佛手), *hehuanpi* (合欢皮) and rose petals or *meiguihua* 玫瑰花. A pleasant herbal tea recipe for calming uses rose and jasmine flowers, which have the actions of soothing the liver and dispersing *qi* stagnation of the liver and thereby alleviating symptoms such as chest tightness, tension and anxiety.

Common prescriptions used in treating depression include *Chaihushugansan* (柴胡疏肝汤) and *Xiaoyaosan* (逍遥散) for alleviating depression associated with blocked *qi* flows in the liver whereas *Ganmaidazao Tang* (甘麦大枣汤) is generally used in blood deficiency syndrome commonly seen in menopausal or post-partum women with frequent mood swings.

Chinese exercises like *qigong* involving breathing, meditation and relaxed movements are thought to promote the flow of *qi* and has traditionally been one way of countering depression. A recent clinical trial involving daily doses of the popular depressant Zoloft against patients taking a walk three times a week showed that the latter gave better therapeutic results.[26] This seems to suggest that the Chinese concept of promoting *qi* flow, through either *qigong* or plain walking exercises, can provide a viable alternative to medications, at least some forms of depression.

12.6 Cancer

The mechanism of growth and spread of cancer cells, after malignant tumours have developed in the body, has been extensively researched, but the underlying reason that cancerous tumours first appear and start to grow in the human body does not appear to be well understood by biomedical science. Certain cancer risk factors have been reasonably well established, such as smoking, environmental pollution, high-fat diets, carcinogens in foods and, in a few cases to specific microbiological agents like the human papilloma virus in cervical cancer and the *Helicobacter pyloris* bacterium in stomach cancer. At a more basic level, inflammation has been associated with the

---

[26] Ilardi, S (2013) Depression as a disease of civilisation. TED talk May 2013.

onset of malignant tumours, as suggested by recent studies. For example, the anti-inflammatory effects of blood serum high density lipoprotein (HDL) were found to be related to lower incidence of cancer.[27]

TCM does not deal with cancer as a disease or a syndrome, and does not have a comprehensive theory explaining the origins of cancer and the principles of therapy for this family of diseases. Chinese medical classics describe conditions that are similar to those found in cancer patients. The *Neijing* states in the *Suwen* that "cough from the lungs, breathlessness and gasping, sometimes even with spitting out of blood....the pallor of the face is floating as with the reverse flow of *qi* (气逆)", likely a depiction of the symptoms of late-stage lung cancer. It attributed the disease to one or more syndromes: toxins in the lung, accumulation of phlegm and dampness in the lungs and deficiency of healthy *qi*.

Breast cancer has been recorded from early historical times. Chao Yuanfang of the Sui dynasty described *Shi Yong* (石痈) as a tumour that "can be felt definitely, with a root. The core and the surface are closely bonding, with slight pain but without heat. It is as hard as a stone." In the Yuan dynasty, Zhu Danxi writing about the disease graphically describes that "the accumulation of depression or anger consumes spleen *qi*, and thus liver *qi* cannot be controlled and is reversed upward to form a tumour like a big chess piece, without pain or itching."[28]

---

[27] Haseeb, J *et al.* (2010) Baseline and on-treatment high-density lipoprotein cholesterol and the risk of cancer in randomized controlled trials of lipid-altering therapy. *Journal of the American College of Cardiology*, 55(25): 2846–2854.

[28] Chao Yuanfang of the Sui dynasty writing in 610 AD about *shi yong* in *The Treatise on the Pathogenesis and Manifestations of All Diseases. Zhu Danxi* (1347 AD) *Ge Zhi Yu Lun (An Inquiry into the Properties of Things).* See Yu and Hong. *Cancer Management with Chinese Medicine.* World Scientific (2012:94).

On the etiology and pathogenesis of breast cancer, Chinese medicine differentiates between the influence of external factors on patients with weak constitutions attacked by the pathogen of wind and cold leading to blood stasis and those of internal emotional factors underlying liver depression with *qi* stagnation harming the spleen and leading to disorders of *qi*, blood circulation and organ functions.[29] From the point of view of TCM theory, the formation of a cancerous tumour, its development and its eventual spread to other parts of the body has its origin in the loss of balance between *yin* and *yang*, manifested in disorders involving the struggle between pathogens and healthy *qi*, and in excess and deficiency syndromes. Such disorders can be brought about by external environmental and internal (emotional and dietary) factors that predispose the body to them.

For the prevention and treatment of cancers, there are lessons to be drawn from Chinese wisdom in *yangsheng*, which revolve around balance and smooth flows in the body achieved through moderation and appropriateness of diet, *qigong* breathing exercises, regularity in living habits, and management of emotions. Even for early-stage cancers of which the patient is deemed cured after medical intervention, there is always a possibility of a relapse if the patient's lifestyle continues to be unhealthy. However the episode of cancer would in most instances have been a wake-up call, spurring the patient to pay more attention to his health, cultivating life somewhat the TCM way: one of regularity in living habits, prudent diet, appropriate exercise and emotional calm, thereby gaining a better chance of long-term freedom from the disease.

To use a social science analogy, we could regard a cancerous tumour as a band of terrorists. After attacking the terrorists

---

[29] *ibid*, 95.

and the initial phase of terrorist activity has been quelled, if the disharmonies of society that bred terrorism in the first place are also resolved and social harmony returns, there is a much better chance of terrorism being truly banished.

12.7 Conclusions

In all the six cases above, TCM provides both complementary and alternative treatments to common chronic illnesses, working largely from the vantage point of restoring imbalances in the body system and encouraging the body's own healing powers to ameliorate symptoms or bring about recovery. It is patient-centric in the sense of addressing directly the nature of the underlying syndromes present and adapting to changing syndromes as the illnesses evolves and progresses in each patient. Despite its ancient origins, TCM has shown remarkable resilience in preserving a healthcare role in modern scientific societies.

13

A Brave New World

Will TCM and biomedicine converge?

In the 21st century, even as TCM clinics and colleges flourish in East Asia and many Western countries, doubts about its scientific credentials persist among a generation of biomedical scientists nurtured in the reductionism of molecular and cellular biology and accustomed to the statistical methods of the so-called 'evidence-based medicine'.

Nevertheless TCM continues to play a significant role in health care worldwide. Among its regular users, the proof of the pudding is in the eating. It enjoys a reputation for healing not demonstrably lower than that of biomedicine. However, the lack of understanding of TCM concepts and methods by biomedical scientists and Western doctors remains an impediment to the appreciation of the potential benefits of incorporating the more familiar and proven parts of TCM into mainstream medicine.

Ironically, a number of Western countries have in a sense gone further in recognising TCM than do some East Asian countries that already have a long tradition in Chinese medicine. In the United States, for example, acupuncture is offered by state-licensed practitioners and eligible for insurance claims. The TCM department at the Cleveland Clinic offers herbal and acupuncture treatments despite acknowledging that many of the therapies lacked sufficient evidence of the kind accepted by modern medicine, but recognising that the continued demand for such treatment by patients may eventually be vindicated by rigorous clinical studies. By contrast, in the former British colonies Hong Kong and Singapore, a strict separation is kept between TCM and Western medicine with very little TCM enjoying state support through clinical or educational services.

Because of the patient-centric nature of TCM emphasising individualised treatment against uniform mass treatment, there is a good case for making more use of observational studies employing reliable patient data from TCM clinics for such studies. Insisting on employing only randomised controlled trials (RCTs) is, to cite a leading expert on evidence-based medicine, being overly narrow in scientific methodology and, more seriously, ignores the limitations of such trials and places them on an 'unwarranted high pedestal'.[30] More recently, the current head of the World Health Organization has challenged the

---

[30] Rawlins, MD (16 October 2008). On the evidence for decisions about the use of therapeutic interventions. Harvein Oration, Royal College of Physicians.

notion that the efficacy of alternative medicine is unproven, and suggested that its usefulness must be evaluated within the more subtle textured context of the culture and environment in which such medicine is practised.[31]

13.1 Modern Medicine and its Discontents

In his acclaimed work *The Rise and Fall of Modern Medicine*, Dr James Le Fanu points out a puzzling paradox. Despite quantum leaps in medical science over the last 60 years since the discovery of the structure of the DNA and dazzling advances in molecular biology, we have failed to answer a basic question of medical science. Le Fanu laments: "Reductionism, the explanation of the phenomena of disease at the most fundamental level of the gene and its products, fails to explain the fact that causes of common diseases are either age-determined or biological and for the most part unknown. Medicine's post-war success, built on the chance discovery of drugs and technological innovation, concealed the fact that its impressive achievements had been won without the necessity to understand the nature or causation of disease. And now medicine still knows the cause of only a fraction of the diseases in the textbooks."[32] Among the diseases that Le Fanu cites are multiple sclerosis, rheumatoid arthritis, schizophrenia, and most forms of cancer.

The idea that most diseases are idiopathic, or of unknown origin, is valid only if we think that only reductionist

---

[31] Dr Margaret Chan, Director-General of the World Health Organization. Opening remarks at the International Forum on Traditional Medicine, China, Macao SAR, 19 August, 2015. http://who.int/dg/speeches/2015/traditional-medicine/en/ (retrieved 29 September 2016).

[32] Le Fanu, J (2011). *The Rise and Fall of Modern Medicine*. New York: Hachette Digital. (The quotation has been slightly edited from several passages on pages 405–495 to read more smoothly.)

explanations make sense. There may be alternative explanations, and TCM provides some of them using holistic models and interpreting human physiology using its own sets of concepts like *qi*, meridians and organs. Diseases are caused by imbalances and disturbed flows in the body, themselves the result of poor living habits as well as environmental and emotional stress. TCM theory, since the time of the publication of the *Neijing*, has argued that modern man changed his lifestyle and diet, which over many millennia had been adapted to man's natural environment. In doing so, the groundwork was laid for illnesses to emerge.

For example, in the TCM framework, a woman with vulnerability to breast cancer has a higher chance of contracting it if she has a high fat diet, lacks exercise, works irregular hours and suffers from prolonged emotional stress that unbalance her body. In holistic TCM medicine, this vulnerability reflects each person's having a constitution that copes less well with a hostile internal and external environment. The only choice for minimising the chance of contracting the disease is to manage these fundamental causal factors. In the biomedical framework terms, a woman's vulnerability to breast cancer may partially be found in a particular gene that raises her likelihood to contract the disease. The gene should not in the TCM framework be regarded the cause of breast cancer. Rather, it is the lifestyle and dietary factors that led her to succumb to this vulnerability.

13.2 *Yangsheng* and the Diseases of Civilisation

The Chinese art of life cultivation or *yangsheng* offers a wealth of insights into the prevention of illness and a rich menu of lifestyle and dietary choices that can restore health to a person with a unhealthy constitution that has not yet developed into a serious disease.

In a dramatic and lucid exposition of the role of lifestyle and diet as the fundamental cause of most chronic illnesses, the American physician Stephen Ilardi postulates that these illnesses as having a common cause, one originating from nothing less than the march of human civilisation itself.[33] In so doing, Ilardi rediscovered the wisdom of the East: these illnesses are the ones that the *Neijing* enjoined us to avoid by following its rules of *yangsheng*. This is the beginning of what is to be hoped the convergence of Western and Chinese medical thought, a return to the basics of disease causation by tracing it to how we conduct our lives.

Ilardi depicts diseases ranging from cancer to depression as 'diseases of civilisation', arguing that Man was evolved in nature with natural foods and a high level of physical activity in daily life. Without electricity and household appliances, daily tasks were done by our hands. Without trains and motor vehicles, our forefathers relied on their feet, keeping their bones, sinews and cardiovascular system in shape. Stress was largely confined to the occasional threat from a wild animal, which would typically be short and intense, lasting for minutes, for which we developed the fight-or-flight response of the sympathetic nervous system. All this was replaced in modern civilisation with processed foods, little exercise other than shortbursts in the gymnasium, and prolonged work and social stresses lasting months and years that wreak havoc on the parasympathetic nervous system.

The solution is to adjust our lifestyles and diets to be as close as possible to those of our forefathers before the industrial

---

[33] Ilardi, S (2013) Depression is a disease of civilization. TED talk May 2013. https://www.youtube.com/watch?v=drv3BP0Fdi8 (retrieved 10 May 2015).

revolution and food processing technology changed our lives and put us at odds with the environment in which our genes evolved over hundreds of generations. Ilardi calls the change in modern living environment 'the radical environment mutation': the environment mutated but our genes have never caught up with it.

Ilardi's prescription for overcoming the diseases of civilisation bears a striking similarity to the injunctions of the *Neijing*: regularity in living habits, moderation in diet, mastery over emotions, exercises that promote *qi* and stimulate smooth flows and balance in the body, and the avoidance of climatic stresses. This paradigm in effect prescribes the attainment of health through lifestyles consistent with our evolutionary origins.

13.3 Longevity and the Ideal Diet

Another vexing problem of modern biomedicine is the ongoing controversy among nutritional scientists over what constitutes a healthy diet. Atkins, Noakes and others advocate a low carbohydrate diet with a relatively high content of animal proteins and unsaturated fat, whilst Campbell and Esselstyn claim epidemiological and clinical evidence for vegetarian diets with high carbohydrate and vegetable protein content.[34] The recent USA government health guidelines suggest that eggs and saturated fat are acceptable in moderate amounts, and challenges the long-held belief that high cholesterol foods result in high blood serum cholesterol. Some modern cardiologists even cast a shade

---

[34]Atkins, RC (2001). *Dr. Atkins' New Diet Revolution Book*, Revised ed. New York: Avon Books. Noakes, T (2014). *The Real Meal Revolution*. Cape Town: Quivertree Publications. Campbell, TC and Campbell, TM (2004). *The China Study*. Dallas: Benbella Books. Esselstyn, CB (2008). *Prevent and Reverse Heart Disease*. New York: Avery.

of doubt on the notion that high serum cholesterol levels increase the risk of cardiovascular disease.[35]

TCM principles may indicate a way out of this messy confusion over diet. TCM prescribes no correct common diet. Diet should be determined by each person's constitution, his living environment and the syndromes that affect him from time to time. The guiding principle is that diet should help him attain *yin-yang* balance and smoothen the flow of *qi* and blood in his body. The old Western aphorism that one man's meat is another man's poison has not lost its relevance for 21st century man. Mongolians led by Genghis Khan wielding swords on horseback and conquering half the civilised world thrived on large amounts of lamb and little vegetable. But their environments and lifestyles over several generations have changed their constitutions and their dietary requirements. Today we witness their weaker descendants riding cars and trains to seek healing at cardiology clinics for their blocked arteries.

Is there a magic common healthy diet for all? If there was, it would contradict one of the tenets of TCM *yangsheng* diet, which calls for adaptation of diet to individual constitutions. This could not have been better validated than by Buettner's study of the 'Blue Zones', regions of the world that boast the highest rate of centenarians.[36] These enclaves of healthy high longevity populations include Sardinian shepherds from Cannonau county who have a high proportion of meat in their diets and drink polyphenol-rich local red wine four times a day. Their men, who do most of the drinking, are exceptional in having a longer average lifespan than their women. Adventists in

---

[35] *New York Times* (2015) http://well.blogs.nytimes.com/2015/02/19/nutrition-panel-callsfor-less-sugar-and-eases-cholesterol-and-fat-restrictions/ (retrieved 29 September 2015).

[36] Buettner, D (2008). *The Blue Zone*. Washington: National Geographic.

California on the other hand thrive on a strict regimen of vegetarian delights and no alcohol. Greeks in the idyllic island of Ikaria feast on the Mediterranean diet rich in olive oil, nuts, vegetables and seafood. And Okinawan centenarians love generous helpings of fat-rich pork with their vegetables. There appears to be no common dietary factor that could account for their longevity.

A conclusion one can draw from the work of scientists like Ilardi and Le Fanu is that reductionist medicine is inadequate for dealing with some of the most fundamental questions of health such as the cause of disease and the right foods to eat. Holistic medicine such as TCM, no matter how abstract its concepts and simplistic its heuristic models, offer alternative views that may well help.

There is hope in the new science of systems biology. This focuses on interactions within biological systems, and is more holistic than reductionist as its principal aim is to model cells and tissues functioning as a system with complex internal networks. This new dimension of biomedical science holds promise in the longer run for a measure of convergence between biomedicine and TCM.

Now we see in part. In time we shall perhaps see the whole:

> For now we see through a glass darkly;
> But then face to face:
> Now I know in part;
> But then I shall know fully.
> (*The Holy Bible: I Corinthians*)

Annex 1: Common Chinese Herbs

Diaphoretic Herbs with Pungent Warm Property 辛温解表药			
Name of Herb	**Flavour and Nature**	**Meridian Tropism**	**Actions**
Mahuang 麻黄 (Ephedra)	Pungent and slightly bitter; Warm	Lung and bladder	1. Induce sweating to relieve superficies 2. Ventilate the lung to relieve asthma 3. Promote diuresis
Guizhi 桂枝 (Cinnamon)	Pungent and sweet; Warm	Heart, lung and bladder	1. Induce sweating to relieve superficies 2. Reinforce *yang* and warm the meridians
Fangfeng 防风 (Divaricate Saposhnikovia Root)	Pungent and sweet; Slightly warm	Bladder, liver and spleen	1. Expel wind 2. Resolve dampness to relieve pain 3. Relieve spasms
Shengjiang 生姜 (Fresh Ginger)	Pungent; Warm	Lung, spleen and stomach	1. Expel wind-cold pathogens 2. Warm the abdomen to relieve nausea and vomiting 3. Warm the lung to relieve cough
Xinyi 辛夷 (Magnolia Biondii Flower)	Pungent; Warm	Lung and stomach	1. Expel wind-cold pathogen 2. Clear the nasal passageway

179

Diaphoretic Herbs with Pungent Cool Property 辛凉解表药

Name of Herb	Flavour and Nature	Meridian Tropism	Actions
Cangerzi 苍耳子 (Siberian Cocklebur Fruit)	Pungent and bitter; Warm; Slightly toxic	Lung	1. Expel wind-cold pathogen 2. Clear the nasal passageway 3. Dispel wind-dampness 4. Relieve pain
Chaihu 柴胡 (Chinese Thorowax Root)	Pungent and bitter; Slightly cold	Liver and gall bladder	1. Relieve exterior syndrome 2. Anti-pyretic 3. Regulate stagnation of liver-*qi* 4. Uplift *yang-qi*
Juhua 菊花 (Chrysanthemum flower)	Pungent, bitter and sweet; Slightly cold	Lung and liver	1. Expel wind-heat 2. Clear liver heat to improve vision 3. Calm and suppress liver-*yang* 4. Eliminate toxins
Sangye 桑叶 (Mulberry Leaf)	Sweet and bitter; Cold	Lung and liver	1. Expel wind-heat 2. Clear lung-heat and nourish dryness 3. Calm and suppress liver-*yang* 4. Clear liver-heat to improve vision
Bohe 薄荷 (Peppermint Leaf)	Pungent; Cool	Lung and liver	1. Expel wind-heat from the head, eye and throat 2. Soothe liver and regulate liver-*qi* stagnation
Gegen 葛根 (Kudzuvine Root)	Pungent and sweet; Cool	Spleen and stomach	1. Anti-pyretic 2. Promote production of fluids to quench thirst 3. Uplift *yang-qi* to stop diarrhoea 4. Promote the outburst of measles

Herbs for Clearing Heat and Purging Fire 清热泻火药

Name of Herb	Flavour and Nature	Meridian Tropism	Actions
Shigao 石膏 (Gypsum)	Sweet and pungent; Very cold	Lung and stomach	Raw form 1. Clear heat and purge fire 2. Remove vexation and quench thirst Calcinated form: Stop bleeding and promote the growth of tissue (for treating ulcers)
Zhimu 知母 (Anemarrhena Rhizome)	Bitter and sweet; Cold	Lung, stomach and kidney	1. Clear heat and purge fire 2. Promote the production of fluids for moistening
Danzhuye 淡竹叶 (Lophatherum Herb)	Sweet and bland; Cold	Heart, stomach and small intestine	1. Clear heat and purge fire 2. Relieve vexation 3. Promote diuresis
Zhizi 栀子 (Cape Jasmine Fruit)	Bitter; Cold	Heart, lung and triple energiser	1. Purge fire to remove vexation 2. Clear heat-dampness 3. Cool the blood and eliminate toxins. Charred form can stop bleeding
Xiakucao 夏枯草 (Common Selfheal Fruit-Spike)	Pungent and bitter; Cold	Liver and gall bladder	1. Clear heart and purge fire to improve vision 2. Disperse abnormal growth/masses to reduce swelling
Juemingzi 决明子 (Cassia Seeds)	Sweet, bitter and salty; Slightly cold	Liver and large intestine	1. Clear liver-heat to improve vision 2. Moisten the large intestine to promote bowel movement

Herbs for Clearing Heat-Dampness 清热燥湿药

Name of Herb	Flavour and Nature	Meridian Tropism	Actions
Huangqin 黄芩 (Baical Skullcap Root/*Radix Scutellariae*)	Bitter; Cold	Lung, gall bladder, spleen, stomach, large and small intestine	1. Clear heat and dry dampness 2. Purge fire and eliminate toxins 3. Stop bleeding 4. Prevent miscarriage
Kushen 苦参 (Light-yellow Sophora Root)	Bitter; Cold	Heart, liver, stomach, large intestine and bladder	1. Clear heat and dry dampness 2. Kill parasites, fungus 3. Promote diuresis

Herbs for Clearing Heat and Eliminating Toxins 清热解毒药

Name of Herb	Flavour and Nature	Meridian Tropism	Actions
Jinyinhua 金银花 (Honeysuckle Flower)	Sweet; Cold	Lung, heart and stomach	1. Eliminate heat and toxins 2. Expel wind-heat pathogens
Lianqiao 连翘 (Weeping Forsythia Capsule)	Bitter; Slightly cold	Lung, heart and small intestine	1. Eliminate heat and toxins 2. Disperse masses/abnormal growth to reduce swelling 3. Expel wind-heat pathogens
Chuanxinlian 穿心莲 (Common Andrographis Herb)	Bitter; Cold	Lung, heart, large intestine and bladder	1. Eliminate heat and toxins 2. Cool the blood 3. Reduce swelling 4. Resolve dampness

(Continued)

(Continued)

Herbs for Clearing Heat and Eliminating Toxins 清热解毒药

Name of Herb	Flavour and Nature	Meridian Tropism	Actions
Banlangen 板蓝根 (Isatis root)	Bitter; Cold	Heart and stomach	1. Eliminate heat and toxins 2. Cool the blood 3. Soothe the throat
Yuxingcao 鱼腥草 (Heartleaf Houttuynia)	Pungent; Slightly cold	Lung	1. Eliminate heat and toxins 2. Reduce abscess by promoting pus discharge 3. Remove dampness by promoting diuresis
Machixian 马齿苋 (Purslane)	Sour; Cold	Liver and large intestine	1. Eliminate heat and toxins 2. Cool the blood to stop bleeding 3. Stop dysentry
Pugongyin 蒲公英 (Dandelion)	Bitter and sweet; Cold	Liver and stomach	1. Eliminate heat and toxins 2. Disperse abnormal growth/masses to reduce swelling 3. Promote diuresis
Banbianlian 半边莲	Pungent; Neutral	Heart, lung and small intestine	1. Eliminate heat and toxins 2. Promote diuresis to relieve edema
Baihua Sheshecao 白花蛇舌草 (Oldenlandia)	Sweet and slightly bitter; Cold	Stomach, large and small intestine	1. Eliminate heat and toxins 2. Remove dampness by promoting diuresis

Heat-Clearing and Blood-Cooling Herbs 清热凉血药

Name of Herb	Flavour and Nature	Meridian Tropism	Actions
Xuanshen 玄参 (Figwort Root)	Sweet, salty and bitter; Slightly cold	Lung, stomach and kidney	1. Clear heat and cool the blood 2. Purge fire and remove toxins 3. Nourish *yin*
Mudanpi 牡丹皮 (Tree Peony Root)	Bitter and sweet; Slightly cold	Heart, liver and kidney	1. Clear heat and cool the blood 2. Promote blood flow and remove stasis
Shengdihuang 生地黄 (Raw Rehmannia Root)	Sweet and bitter; Cold	Heart, liver and kidney	1. Clear heat and cool the blood 2. Nourish *yin* and promote the production of fluids

Herbs for Clearing Asthenic Heat 清虚热药

Name of Herb	Flavour and Nature	Meridian Tropism	Actions
Qinghao 青蒿 (Sweet wormwood)	Bitter and pungent; Cold	Liver and gall bladder	1. Clear asthenic heat and summer heat 2. Cool the blood 3. Treat malaria

Purgatives 泻下药

Name of Herb	Flavour and Nature	Meridian Tropism	Actions
Dahuang 大黄 (Rhubarb)	Bitter; Cold	Spleen, stomach, large intestine, liver and pericardium	1. Promote bowel movement by clearing heat and purging fire 2. Cool blood and remove toxins 3. Remove blood stasis
Fanxieye 番泻叶 (Senna Leaf)	Sweet and bitter; Cold	Large intestine	Purge to promote bowel movement
Huomaren 火麻仁 (Hemp Seed)	Sweet; Neutral	Spleen, stomach and large intestine	Promote bowel movement by moistening the intestine

Herbs for Resolving Dampness 化湿药

Name of Herb	Flavour and Nature	Meridian Tropism	Actions
Huoxiang 藿香 (Cablin Patchouli Herb)	Pungent; Slightly warm	Spleen, stomach and lung	1. Resolve dampness 2. Relieve nausea and vomiting 3. Clear summer-heat
Cangzhu 苍术 (Atractylodes Rhizome)	Pungent and bitter; Warm	Spleen, stomach and liver	1. Dry dampness and strengthen the spleen 2. Expel wind and disperse the cold
Houpo 厚朴 (Officinal Magnolia Bark)	Pungent and bitter; Warm	Spleen, stomach, lung and large intestine	1. Dry dampness and resolve phlegm 2. Promote the descent of *qi* to remove stagnation
Sharen 砂仁 (Villous Amomum Fruit)	Pungent; Warm	Spleen, stomach and kidney	1. Resolve dampness and regulate *qi* 2. Warm the abdomen and stop diarrhoea 3. Prevent miscarriage
Doukou 豆蔻 (Cardamon Fruit)	Pungent; Warm	Spleen, stomach and lung	1. Resolve dampness and regulate *qi* 2. Warm the abdomen to relieve nausea and vomiting

Herbs for Removing Wind-Dampness 祛风湿药

Name of Herb	Flavour and Nature	Meridian Tropism	Actions
Wujiapi 五加皮 (Slenderstyle Acanthopanax Bark)	Pungent and bitter; Warm	Liver and kidney	1. Remove wind-dampness 2. Tonify the liver and kidney 3. Strengthen the ligaments and bone 4. Promote diuresis

Diuretics 利水渗湿药

Name of Herb	Flavour and Nature	Meridian Tropism	Actions
Fuling 茯苓 (Poria)	Sweet and bland; Neutral	Heart, spleen and kidney	1. Promote diuresis to drain dampness and relieve edema 2. Invigorate spleen 3. Tranquilise the mind
Yiyiren 薏苡仁 (Job's Tears)	Sweet and bland; Cool	Spleen, stomach and lung	1. Promote diuresis to drain dampness and relieve edema 2. Invigorate spleen 3. Relieve joint pain 4. Clear heat and promote pus discharge
Dongguaren 冬瓜仁 (Winter melon seeds)	Sweet; Cool	Spleen and small intestine	1. Clear lung-heat and resolve phlegm 2. Remove dampness and promote pus discharge

Herbs for Regulating *Qi* 理气药

Name of Herb	Flavour and Nature	Meridian Tropism	Actions
Chenpi 陈皮 (Dried tangerine peel)	Pungent and bitter; Warm	Spleen and lung	1. Regulate *qi* and invigorate spleen 2. Dry dampness and resolve phlegm
Xiangfu 香附 (Nutgrass Galingale Rhizome)	Pungent, slightly bitter and sweet; Neutral	Liver, spleen and triple energiser	1. Regulate liver-*qi* stagnation 2. Regulate menstruation and relieve pain 3. Regulate spleen and stomach-*qi*
Meiguihua 玫瑰花 (Rose flower)	Sweet and slightly bitter; Warm	Spleen and liver	1. Regulate liver-*qi* stagnation 2. Promote blood flow to relieve pain

Herbs for Promoting Digestion 消食药

Name of Herb	Flavour and Nature	Meridian Tropism	Actions
Shanzha 山楂 (Hawthorn Berry)	Sweet and sour; Slightly warm	Spleen, stomach and liver	1. Promote digestion 2. Regulate *qi* and remove stasis
Maiya 麦芽 (Germinated Barley)	Sweet; Neutral	Spleen, stomach and liver	1. Promote digestion and strengthen the stomach 2. Relieve breast engorgement. Stop lactation.
Laifuzi 莱菔子 (Radish seed)	Sweet and pungent; Neutral	Spleen, stomach and lung	1. Promote digestion and relieve abdomen distension 2. Promote the descent of *qi* and resolve dampness

Interior Warming Herbs 温里药

Name of Herb	Flavour and Nature	Meridian Tropism	Actions
Fuzi 附子 (Lateralis Preparata)	Pungent and sweet; Very Hot;Toxic	Heart, spleen and kidney	1. Restore *yang* (for severe deficiency of *yang*) 2. Strengthen *yang* by restoring fire 3. Disperse cold to alleviate pain
Ganjiang 干姜 (Zingiber Dried Ginger)	Pungent; Hot	Spleen, stomach, kidney, heart and lung	1. Warm the abdomen and disperse cold 2. Restore *yang* to warm and clear the collaterals 3. Warm the lung to resolve rheum
Rougui 肉桂 (Cassia Bark)	Pungent and sweet; Very Hot	Kidney, spleen, heart and liver	1. Strengthen *yang* by restoring fire 2. Disperse cold to alleviate pain 3. Warm the meridians to clear the collaterals 4. Return fire to the origin (kidney)
Huajiao 花椒 (Pricklyash Peel)	Pungent; Warm	Spleen, stomach and kidney	1. Warm the abdomen to relieve pain 2. Kill parasites to relieve itching

Hemostatics 止血药

Name of Herb	Flavour and Nature	Meridian Tropism	Actions
Sanqi 三七	Sweet and slightly bitter; Warm	Liver and stomach	1. Remove blood stasis to stop bleeding 2. Promote blood circulation to relieve pain

Herbs for Promoting Blood Circulation and Removing Stasis 活血化瘀药

Name of Herb	Flavour and Nature	Meridian Tropism	Actions
Chuanxiong 川芎 (Szechwan Lovage Rhizome)	Pungent; Warm	Liver, gall bladder and pericardium	1. Promote blood circulation and regulate *qi* 2. Expel wind to relieve pain
Jianghuang 姜黄 (Tumeric)	Pungent and bitter; Warm	Spleen and liver	1. Promote blood circulation and regulate *qi* 2. Clear the collaterals to relieve pain
Moyao 没药 (Myrrh)	Pungent and bitter; Neutral	Heart, liver and spleen	1. Promote blood circulation to relieve pain 2. Reduce swelling and promote healing
Danshen 丹参	Bitter; Slightly cold	Heart, pericardium, and liver	1. Promote blood circulation to regulate menstruation 2. Remove stasis to relieve pain 3. Cool the blood to promote the healing of carbuncle 4. Remove vexation and calm the mind
Taoren 桃仁 (Peach Seed)	Bitter and sweet; Neutral; Slightly toxic	Heart, liver and large intestine	1. Promote blood circulation and remove stasis 2. Moisten the large intestine to promote bowel movement 3. Relieve cough and dyspnea
Honghua 红花 (Safflower)	Pungent; Warm	Heart and liver	1. Promote blood circulation and menstruation 2. Remove blood stasis to relieve pain

Herbs for Resolving Phlegm and Relieving Cough and Dyspnea 止咳化痰平喘药

Name of Herb	Flavour and Nature	Meridian Tropism	Actions
Banxia 半夏 (Pinellia Tuber)	Pungent; Warm; Toxic	Spleen, stomach and lung	1. Dry dampness and resolve phlegm 2. Relieve nausea and vomiting by suppressing the adverse rise of *qi* 3. Relieve abdominal distension and disperse masses
Jiegeng 桔梗 (Hogfennel Root)	Bitter and pungent; Neutral	Lung	1. Disperse lung-*qi* 2. Expel phlegm 3. Soothe the throat 4. Promote the discharge of pus
Gualou 瓜蒌 (Snakegourd Fruit)	Sweet and slightly bitter; Cold	Lung, stomach and large intestine	1. Clear heat and resolve phlegm 2. Regulate *qi* stagnation in the chest and disperse abnormal masses/growths 3. Moisten the large intestine to promote bowel movement
Chuanbeimu 川贝母 (Tendrilleaf Fritillary Bulb)	Bitter and Sweet; Slightly cold	Lung and heart	1. Clear heat and resolve phlegm 2. Moisten the lung to relieve cough 3. Disperse abnormal masses or growths to reduce swelling
Zhebeimu 浙贝母 (Thunberg Fritillary Bulb)	Bitter; Cold	Lung and heart	1. Clear heat and resolve phlegm 2. Disperse abnormal masses or growths to promote healing of carbuncle

(Continued)

(Continued)

Herbs for Resolving Phlegm and Relieving Cough and Dyspnea 止咳化痰平喘 药

Name of Herb	Flavour and Nature	Meridian Tropism	Actions
Luohanguo 罗汉果	Sweet; Cool	Lung and large intestine	1. Clear heat from the lung and soothe the throat 2. Resolve phlegm and relieve cough 3. Moisten the large intestine to promote bowel movement
Kuxingren 苦杏仁 (Bitter Almond Seed)	Bitter; Slightly warm; Slightly toxic	Lung and large intestine	1. Relieve cough and dyspnea 2. Moisten the large intestine to promote bowel movement
Ziyuan 紫菀 (Tatarian Aster Root)	Bitter, sweet and pungent; Slightly warm	Lung	1. Moisten the lung and resolve phlegm to relieve cough
Kuandonghua 款冬花 (Common Clotsfoot Flower)	Pungent and slightly bitter; Warm	Lung	1. Moisten the lung, promote the descending of lung-qi and resolve phlegm to relieve cough
Pipaye 枇杷叶 (Loquat Leaf)	Bitter; Slightly cold	Lung and stomach	1. Clear lung heat to relieve cough 2. Promote the descent of qi to relieve nausea and vomiting
Baiguo 白果 (Gingko Seed)	Sweet, bitter and astringent; Neutral; Toxic	Lung	1. Astringe lung and resolve phlegm to relieve dyspnea 2. Stop abnormal vagina discharge (leucorrhoea) and reduce urination

	Calmatives 安神药		
Name of Herb	**Flavour and Nature**	**Meridian Tropism**	**Actions**
Longgu 龙骨 (Dragon Bone)	Sweet and astringent; Neutral	Heart, lung and kidney	1. Tranquilise the mind 2. Calm the liver to suppress liver-*yang* 3. Arrest fluids (calcinated form)
Suanzaoren 酸枣仁 (Spine Date Seed)	Sour and sweet; Neutral	Heart, liver and gall bladder	1. Nourish the heart and liver 2. Calm the mind 3. Arrest sweating
Yejiaoteng 夜交藤	Sweet; Neutral	Heart and liver	1. Nourish the blood to calm the mind 2. Expel wind to clear the collaterals
Baiziren 柏子仁 (Chinese Arborvitae Kernel)	Sweet; Neutral	Heart, kidney and large intestine	1. Nourish the heart to calm the mind 2. Moisten the intestine to promote bowel movement
Hehuanpi 合欢皮 (Silktree Albizia Bark)	Sweet; Neutral	Heart, liver and lung	1. Alleviate depression to calm the mind 2. Promote blood circulation to relieve swelling
Lingzhi 灵芝 (Lucid Ganoderma)	Sweet; Neutral	Heart, lung, liver and kidney	1. Strengthen *qi* to calm the mind 2. Relieve cough and asthma

Qi Tonics 补气药

Name of Herb	Flavour and Nature	Meridian Tropism	Actions
Renshen 人参 (Ginseng)	Sweet, Slightly bitter; Neutral	Lung, spleen and heart	1. Invigorate *qi* 2. Tonify the spleen and strengthen the lung 3. Promote the production of fluids 4. Calm the nerves for better concentration and also sounder sleep
Xiyangshen 西洋参 (American Ginseng)	Sweet, Slightly bitter; Cool	Lung, heart, kidney and spleen	1. Invigorate *qi* and nourish *yin* 2. Clear heat and promote the production of fluids
Dangshen 党参 (Tangshen)	Sweet; Neutral	Spleen and lung	1. Invigorate the spleen and lung functions by tonifying their *qi* 2. Tonify blood 3. Promote the production of fluids
Taizishen 太子参 (Heterophylly Falsestarwort Root)	Sweet, Slightly bitter; Neutral	Spleen and lung	1. Invigorate *qi* and strengthen the spleen functions 2. Promote the production of fluids to moisten the lung
Huangqi 黄芪 (Astragalus)	Sweet; Slightly warm	Spleen and lung	1. Strengthen the spleen functions 2. Uplift *yang-qi* 3. Consolidate the exterior to strengthen the body's defence against external pathogens 4. Promote diuresis and the healing of wounds/ ulcers

(Continued)

(*Continued*)

Qi Tonics 补气药

Name of Herb	Flavour and Nature	Meridian Tropism	Actions
Baizhu 白术 (Largehead Astractylodes Rhizome)	Sweet and bitter; Warm	Spleen and stomach	1. Strengthen spleen and tonify *qi* 2. Dry dampness and promote diuresis 3. Stop perspiration 4. Prevent miscarriage
Shanyao 山药 (Wild Yam)	Sweet; Neutral	Spleen, lung and kidney	1. Tonify the spleen and nourish the stomach 2. Promote the production of fluids and tonify the lung 3. Tonify the kidney 4. Conserve essence
Gancao 甘草 (Liquorice Root)	Sweet; Neutral	Heart, lung, spleen and stomach	1. Tonify the spleen 2. Resolve phlegm and relieve cough 3. Relieve pain 4. Clear heat and eliminate toxins (raw liquorice) 5. Regulate the actions of herbs in a prescription
Dazao 大枣 (Chinese Dates)	Sweet; Warm	Spleen, stomach and heart	1. Strengthen the spleen functions and tonify *qi* 2. Nourish blood to calm the mind
Baibiandou 白扁豆 (White Hyacinth Bean)	Sweet; Slightly Warm	Spleen and stomach	1. Tonify the spleen 2. Resolve dampness

Yang Tonics 补阳药

Name of Herb	Flavour and Nature	Meridian Tropism	Actions
Lurong 鹿茸 (Hairy Antler)	Sweet and salty; Warm	Kidney and lung liver	1. Tonify kidney-*yang* 2. Tonify blood and essence 3. Strengthen the bone and tendons 4. Regulate the *chong* 冲 and *ren* 任 vessels (they govern the menstruation) 5. Promote the healing of sores/ulcers
Yinyanghuo 淫羊藿 (Horny-goat Weed)	Pungent and sweet; Warm	Kidney and liver	1. Tonify the kidney and boost *yang* 2. Expel wind and remove dampness
Duzhong 杜仲 (Eucommia Bark)	Sweet; Warm	Liver and kidney	1. Tonify the kidney and liver 2. Strengthen the bones and tendons 3. Prevent miscarriage
Dongchongxiacao 冬虫夏草 (Cordyceps)	Sweet and salty; Warm	Kidney and lung	1. Tonify the kidney and lung 2. Resolve phlegm 3. Stop bleeding
Hetaoren 核桃仁 (Walnut)	Sweet; Warm	Kidney, lung and large intestine	1. Tonify the kidney and warm the lung 2. Moisten the large intestine to promote bowel movement

Blood Tonics 补血药

Name of Herb	Flavour and Nature	Meridian Tropism	Actions
Shudihuang 熟地黄 (Processed Rehmannia Root)	Sweet; Slightly warm	Liver and kidney	1. Tonify blood and nourish *yin* 2. Supplement essence and marrow
Ejiao 阿胶 (Equus asinus Linnaeus)	Sweet; Neutral	Lung, liver and kidney	1. Tonify blood and nourish *yin* 2. Moisten the lung 3. Stop bleeding
Heshouwu 何首乌 (Fleeceflower Root)	Bitter, sweet, astringent; Slightly warm	Kidney and liver	Processed form: 1. Tonify and enrich blood Raw form: 1. Eliminate toxins 2. Treat malaria 3. Moisten the large intestine to promote bowel movement
Longyanrou 龙眼肉 (Logan Meat)	Sweet; Warm	Heart and spleen	1. Tonify the heart and spleen 2. Nourish blood to calm the mind
Danggui 当归 (Chinese Angelica)	Sweet and pungent; Warm	Liver, heart and spleen	1. Tonify blood and regulate menstruation 2. Promote blood circulation to relieve pain 3. Moisten the large intestine to promote bowel movement

Yin Tonics 补阴药

Name of Herb	Flavour and Nature	Meridian Tropism	Actions
Beishashen 北沙参 (Coastal Glehnia Root)	Sweet and slightly bitter; Slightly cold	Lung and stomach	1. Nourish lung-*yin* and clear lung heat 2. Tonify the stomach and promote the production of fluids
Baihe 百合 (Lily Bulb)	Sweet; Slightly cold	Lung, heart and stomach	1. Nourish *yin* and moisten the lung 2. Clear heat from the heart to calm the mind
Maidong 麦冬 (Dwarf Lilyturf Tuber)	Sweet and slightly bitter; Slightly cold	Lung, stomach and heart	1. Nourish *yin* and promote the production of fluids 2. Moisten the lung 3. Clear heat from the heart
Shihu 石斛 (Dendrobium)	Sweet; Slightly cold	Stomach and kidney	1. Tonify the stomach and promote the production of fluids 2. Nourish *yin* and clear asthenic heat
Yuzhu 玉竹 (Fragrant Solomonseal Rhizome)	Sweet; Slightly cold	Lung and stomach	1. Nourish *yin* and moisten dryness 2. Promote the production of fluids to quench thirst
Gouqizi 枸杞子 (Wolfberry Seed)	Sweet; Neutral	Liver and kidney	1. Nourish and tonify the kidney and liver 2. Tonify essence and improve vision
Guijia 龟甲 (Tortise Shell)	Sweet and salty; Cold	Liver, kidney and heart	1. Nourish *yin* and suppress *yang* 2. Tonify kidney and strengthen bone 3. Nourish blood and tonify the heart
Heizhima 黑芝麻 (Black Sesame Seed)	Sweet; Neutral	Liver, kidney and large intestine	1. Tonify the kidney and liver 2. Moisten the large intestine 3. Tonify essence and blood

Astringent Herbs 收涩药

Name of Herb	Flavour and Nature	Meridian Tropism	Actions
Wuweizi 五味子 (Chinese Magnoliavine Fruit)	Sour and sweet; Slightly warm	Lung, heart and kidney	1. Reduce sweating 2. Calm the mind 3. Tonify the kidney 4. Tonify *qi* and promote the production of fluids
Lianzi 莲子 (Lotus seed)	Sweet and astringent; Neutral	Spleen, heart and kidney	1. Prevent abnormal discharge and involuntary seminal emission 2. Tonify the spleen to relieve diarrhoea 3. Tonify the kidney 4. Calm the mind by nourishing the heart

Annex 2: Common Chinese Prescriptions

The prescriptions listed below are representative of the various formulations categorised by their principal therapeutic functions. The Chinese names are provided and, where commonly used, the English translations as well. Each prescription typically ends with 'san' if it is usually prepared as a powder, 'yin' or 'tang' if it is a decoction and 'wan' if in pill form. In practice, most decoctions are also available in pharmacies in the form of pills, tablets or capsules as these are more convenient for daily use.

Diaphoretic Prescriptions		
1	Yinqiaosan 银翘散	Expels wind-heat exogenous pathogens. Eliminates heat and toxins. Often used in the early stage of an external syndrome invaded by wind-heat pathogens.
2	Guizhitang 桂枝汤	Expels wind-cold exogenous pathogens. Regulates the nutrient and defensive *qi* to strengthen the body. Can be used for treating external syndromes caused by wind-cold exogenous pathogens or for individuals who feel weak and are recovering from chronic illnesses.

(Continued)

(Continued)

	Prescriptions for Clearing Internal Heat	
3	Daochisan 导赤散	Clears heat from the heart. Promotes diuresis and nourishes *yin*. Treats the syndrome of exuberance of heart fire.
4	Longdan Xiegan Tang 龙胆泻肝汤	Purges fire from the liver and gall bladder. Clears dampness and heat in the lower energiser. Treats sthenic syndrome of the exuberance of liver fire.
5	Yunujian 玉女煎	Clears heat from the stomach and nourishes kidney-*yin*. Treats the syndrome of stomach fire with *yin* deficiency.
	Prescriptions for Removing Dampness	
6	Huoxiang Zhengqi San 藿香正气散	Removes dampness and regulates *qi* in the abdomen region. Used for treating vomiting and diarrhoea caused by cold dampness and wind.
7	Wulingsan 五苓散	Promotes diuresis and removes dampness. Warms *yang-qi* to enhance the function of *qi* to regulate water metabolism. Can be used for treating edema due to retention of water and dampness.
	Prescriptions for Removing Wind-Dampness	
8	Duhuo Jisheng Tang 独活寄生汤	Expels wind-dampness to relieve arthritic pain. Tonifies kidney, liver, *qi* and blood. Treats deficiency syndrome in liver, kidney, *qi* and blood.
9	Danggui Niantong Tang 当归拈痛汤	Drains dampness and clears heat. Expels wind to relieve arthritic pain. Treats damp-heat syndrome.
10	Juanbitang 蠲痹汤	Tonifies *qi* and nourishes blood. Expels wind and dampness. Treats wind-cold-dampness syndrome and relieves arthritic pain.

(Continued)

(Continued)

	Prescriptions for Promoting Digestion	
11	Baohewan 保和丸 'Pill for Preserving Harmony'	Promotes digestion of food. Treats food retention syndrome.
	Prescriptions for Promoting Blood Flow and Removing Blood Stasis	
12	Xuefu Zhuyu Tang 血府逐瘀汤	Promotes blood flow and removes stasis. Regulates *qi* and relieves pain. Often used for treating blood stasis syndrome.
	Prescriptions for Resolving Phlegm and Relieving Cough	
13	Qingqi Huatan Tang 清气化痰汤	Clears heat and resolves phlegm. Regulates *qi* and relieves cough. Treats heat-phlegm syndrome.
14	Banxia Houpo Tang 半夏厚朴汤	Regulates *qi* to disperse clumps. Suppresses adverse rise of *qi* and resolves phlegm. Treats 梅核气 *meiheqi* — a feeling of something in the throat that cannot be swallowed or expectorated.
15	Erchen Tang 二陈汤	Removes dampness, resolves phlegm and promotes *qi* flow. Used in wet cough due to phlegm-dampness with white sputum.
	Prescriptions for Calming the Mind	
16	Suanzaoren Tang 酸枣仁汤 'Jujube Seed Decoction'	Nourishes blood and calms the mind. Clears asthenic heat to relieve vexation. Often used to treat insomnia resulting from the deficiency syndrome in liver blood.
17	Tianwang Buxin Dan 天王补心丹	Nourishes *yin* and blood. Tranquilises heart to calm the mind. Treats *yin* deficiency syndrome in the heart and kidney.

(Continued)

(Continued)

	Prescriptions for Regulating the Liver and Spleen	
18	Xiaoyao San 逍遥散 'Ease Powder'	Soothes the liver and regulates the spleen. Used in stagnation of liver-*qi* and deficiency of blood and spleen, with liver suppressing spleen (over-restraint relationship).
19	Danzhi Xiaoyaosan 丹栀逍遥散 (extension of ease powder)	Soothes the liver, regulates *qi* and clears liver fire. Used in liver stagnation stirring up fire.
	Prescriptions for Removing Wind (Both Exogenous and Endogenous Wind)	
20	Tianma Gouteng Yin 天麻钩藤饮	Calms the liver to remove endogenous wind. Clears heat and nourishes liver/kidney. Used for treating headache and dizziness caused by hyperactivity of liver-*yang* syndrome.
21	Xiaofengsan 消风散	Expels wind and nourishes blood. Clears heat and removes dampness. Treats eczema and rubella caused by wind-heat or wind-dampness syndrome.
	Prescriptions for Removing Dryness	
22	Qingzao Jiufei Tang 清燥救肺汤	Clears exogenous dry-heat pathogen and moistens the lung. Treats severe syndrome of dryness in the lung.
23	Baihe Gujing Tang 百合固金汤	Nourishes *yin* and moistens lung. Resolves phlegm and relieves cough. Treats cough caused by the deficiency syndrome of kidney and lung-*yin*. (Used in the more advanced stage as the lung-*yin* has been severely damaged.)

(Continued)

(Continued)

	Prescriptions for Tonifying *Qi*	
24	Decoction of the Four Noble Herbs (Sijunzi Tang) 四君子汤	Tonifies *qi* and strengthens spleen. Used in deficiency syndrome of spleen and stomach.
25	Decoction of the Six Noble Herbs 六君子汤 (extension of Decoction of the Four Noble Herbs)	Used for deficiency of spleen/stomach syndrome with dampness and phlegm.
26	Decoction of *Xiangsha Liujunzi Tang* 香砂六君子汤 (extension of Decoction of Six Noble Herbs)	Used for spleen-stomach deficiency with more pronounced dampness and phlegm leading to *qi* stagnation.
27	Shenling Baizhu San 参苓白术散	Tonifies *qi* and strengthens spleen. Resolves dampness. Treats *qi* deficiency syndrome of the spleen and stomach with dampness.
28	Buzhong Yiqi Tang 补中益气汤	Tonifies *qi* and strengthens spleen. Uplifts spleen *yang-qi*. Treats *qi* deficiency syndrome of the spleen and stomach.
29	Yupingfeng San 玉屏风散 (Jade Screen Powder)	Replenishes *qi*, consolidates the superficies and arrests perspiration (reduces sweating). Used in individuals with *qi* deficiency (defensive *qi*).

(Continued)

(Continued)

30	Pulse-activating Powder 生脉饮 (*Shengmai Yin*)	Tonifies *qi* and promotes the production of fluids. Astringes *yin* and arrests sweating. For treatment of deficiency syndrome of *qi* and *yin* resulting in spontaneous sweating and chronic dry cough accompanied by breathlessness, fatigue, etc.
Prescriptions for Tonifying Blood		
31	Decoction of the Four Ingredients 四物汤 (*Siwu Tang*)	Nourishes and regulates blood without introducing stasis. Used in blood deficiency syndrome; Often used for regulating menstruation.
32	Decoction of *Taohong Siwu Tang* 桃红四物汤 (extension of decoction of the four ingredients)	Promotes blood circulation and removes stasis. Used in blood deficiency syndrome with stasis resulting in early menses with blood clots.
33	Chinese Angelica Decoction for Tonifying the Blood 当归补血汤 (Danggui Buxue Tang)	Invigorates *qi* to promote blood production. Used in blood deficiency syndrome, particularly blood deficiency with fever and headache following childbirth or menstrual disorder with severe loss of blood; anemia.
34	Decoction for Restoring the Spleen 归脾汤 (*Guipitang*)	Tonifies *qi* and blood. Strengthens the spleen and nourishes the heart. Treats deficiency syndrome in heart and spleen.
35	Danggui Yinzi 当归饮子	Nourishes blood and promotes its flow. Expels wind to relieve pain. Treats eczema or rubella caused by blood deficiency syndrome (with the invasion of wind pathogen).

(Continued)

(Continued)

Prescriptions for Tonifying *Qi* and Blood		
36	Decoction of the 8 Precious Ingredients 八珍汤	Nourishes *qi* and blood. Used for those with prolonged weakness of *qi* and blood caused by excessive haemorrhage and low *qi* level.
37	Shiquan Dabutang 十全大补汤 'Decoction of 10 Powerful Herbs' (extension of decoction of the 8 precious ingredients)	Warms and tonifies *qi* and blood. Used in deficiency syndrome in *qi* and blood, accompanied by slight *yang* deficiency.
Prescriptions for Tonifying Yang		
38	Pill for Nourishing Kidney-*Yang* (Shenqi Wan) 肾气丸	Warms and invigorates kidney-*yang*. Used to treat deficiency of kidney-*yang* syndrome, often accompanied by weakness of back and knees, coldness in lower trunk, frequent night urination, sexual dysfunction.
39	Jisheng Shenqi Wan 济生肾气丸 (extension of Shenqi Wan)	Warms kidney-*yang* and promotes diuresis to relieve edema. It is often used to treat water retention due to kidney-*yang* deficiency.
Prescriptions for Tonifying Yin		
40	Liuwei Dihuang Wan 六味地黄丸 'Pill of Six Ingredients with Rehmanniae'	Nourishes *yin* and invigorates the kidney. Used in deficiency syndrome of kidney and liver-*yin*, leading to flare up of kidney deficiency fire. Marked by tinnitus, night sweats, emissions, sore throat. Some diabetes patients exhibit such a syndrome.

3

Glossary of Common Names of Herbs

Chinese Name	中文名	Common Name in English
	A	
Aiye	艾叶	Argy wormwood leaf
	B	
Baibiandou	白扁豆	White hyacinth bean
Baibu	百部	Stemona root
Baifan	白矾	Alum
Baifuzi	白附子	White aconite root
Baihe	百合	Lily bulb

(Continued)

(Continued)

Chinese Name	中文名	Common Name in English
Baiji	白及	Common bletilla tuber
Baimuer	白木耳	White fungus
Baishao	白芍	White peony root
Baixianpi	白鲜皮	Densefruit pittany root-bark
Baizhi	白芷	Dahurian angelica root
Baizhu	白术	Largehead atractylodes rhizome
Baiziren	柏子仁	Chinese arborvitae kernel
Bajitian	巴戟天	Morinda root
Banlangen	板蓝根	Isatis root
Banxia	半夏	Pinellia tuber
Beishashen	北沙参	Coastal glehnia root
Bingpian	冰片	Bomeol
Binlang	槟榔	Areca seed
Bohe	薄荷	Peppermint
Buguzhi	补骨脂	Malaytea scurfpea fruit
	C	
Cangerzi	苍耳子	Siberian cocklebur fruit
Cangzhu	苍术	Atractylodes rhizome
Caowu	草乌	Kusnezoff monkshood root
Cebaiye	侧柏叶	Chinese arborvitac twig and leaf
Chaihu	柴胡	Chinese thorowax root
Chantui	蝉蜕	Cicada slough
Chenpi	陈皮	Dried tangerine peel
Chenxiang	沉香	Chinese eaglewood
Cheqianzi	车前子	Plantain seed
Chishao	赤芍	Red peony root
Chishizhi	赤石脂	Red halloysite

(Continued)

(Continued)

Chinese Name	中文名	Common Name in English
Chixiaodou	赤小豆	Red beans
Chuaniuxi	川牛膝	Medicinal cyathula root
Chuanlianzi	川楝子	Sichuan chinaberry fruit
Chuanshanjia	穿山甲	Pangolin scale
Chuanwu	川乌	Common monkshood mother root
Chuanxiong	川芎	Szechwan lovage rhizome
D		
Dafupi	大腹皮	Areca peel
Dahuang	大黄	Rhubarb
Danggui	当归	Chinese angelica root
Dangshen	党参	Codonopsis root
Dannanxing	胆南星	Bile arisaema
Danshen	丹参	Red sage root
Daqingye	大青叶	Dyers woad leaf
Dazao	大枣	Chinese date
Dazhuye	淡竹叶	Lophathrum herb
Difuzi	地肤子	Belvedere fruit
Digupi	地骨皮	Chinese wolfberry root-bark
Dihuang	地黄	Rehmannia root
Dilong	地龙	Ground dragon
Diyu	地榆	Garden burnet root
Doukou	豆蔻	Round cardamon fruit
Duhuo	独活	Doubleteeth pubescent angelica root
Duzhong	杜仲	Eucommia bark
E		
Ejiao	阿胶	Gelatin
Ezhu	莪术	Zedoray rhizome

(Continued)

(Continued)

Chinese Name	中文名	Common Name in English
F		
Fabanxia	法半夏	Pinellia tuber processed with radix glycyrrhizae and lime
Fangfeng	防风	Divaricate saposhnikvia root
Fangji	防己	Fourstamen stephania root
Fengfang	蜂房	Honeycomb
Foshou	佛手	Finger citron
Fuling	茯苓	Poria/Indian bread
Fupenzi	覆盆子	Chinese raspberry
Fuxiaomai	浮小麦	Unripe wheat grain
G		
Gancao	甘草	Liquorice root
Ganjiang	干姜	Dried ginger
Gaolishen	高丽参	Korean ginseng
Gegen	葛根	Kudzuvine root
Gouqizi	枸杞子	Barbary wolfberry fruit
Gouteng	钩藤	Gambir plant
Gualou	瓜蒌	Snake gourd fruit
Guijia	龟甲	Tortise shell
Guizhi	桂枝	Cassia twig
Guya	谷芽	Millet sprout
H		
Haipiaoxiao	海螵蛸	Cuttlebone
Hanliancao	旱莲草	Eclipta/Yerbadetajo herb
Hehuanhua	合欢花	Albizia flower
Hehuanpi	合欢皮	Silktree albizia bark
Heimuer	黑木耳	Black fungus

(Continued)

(Continued)

Chinese Name	中文名	Common Name in English
Heshouwu	何首乌	Fleeceflower root
Heye	荷叶	Lotus leaf
Honghua	红花	Safflower
Houpo	厚朴	Officinal magnolia bark
Huaijiao	槐角	Japanese pagodatree pod
Huaishan	淮山	Chinese yam
Huajiao	花椒	Prickly ash peel
Huangbai	黄柏	Amur cork-tree
Huangjing	黄精	Solomonseal rhizome
Huanglian	黄连	Golden thread
Huangqi	黄芪	Milkvetch root
Huangqin	黄芩	Baical skullcap root
Huashi	滑石	Talc
Huhuanglian	胡黄连	Figwortflower picrorhiza rhizome
Huoxiang	藿香	Cablin patchouli herb
Huzhang	虎杖	Giant Knotweed rhizome

J

Jiegeng	桔梗	Platycodon root
Jili	蒺藜	Puncturevine caltrop fruit
Jineijin	鸡内金	Chicken's gizzard skin
Jingjie	荆芥	Fineleaf schizonepeta herb
Jinmaogouji	金毛狗脊	Chain fern rhizome
Jinzhencai	金针菜	Dried Lily flower
Jixueteng	鸡血藤	Suberect spatholobus stem
Juhong	橘红	Red tangerine peel
Juhua	菊花	Chrysanthemum flower
Juiyinhua	金银花	Honeysuckle flower

(Continued)

(Continued)

Chinese Name	中文名	Common Name in English
	K	
Kuandonghua	款冬花	Common coltsfoot flower
Kushen	苦参	Lightyellow sophora root
Kuxingren	苦杏仁	Bitter apricot seed
	L	
Lianqiao	连翘	Weeping forsythia gapsule
Lianzi	莲子	Lotus seed
Longdancao	龙胆草	Chinese gentian
Longyanrou	龙眼肉	Longan aril
Luhui	芦荟	Aloes
Lulutong	路路通	Sweet gum fruit
	M	
Machixian	马齿苋	Purslane herb
Mahuang	麻黄	Ephedra
Maidong	麦冬	Dwarf lilyturf tuber
Maiya	麦芽	Germinated barley
Mingdangshen	明党参	Medicinal changium root
Mudanpi	牡丹皮	Tree peony bark
Muli	牡蛎	Oyster shell
Muxiang	木香	Costus root
	N	
Niubangzi	牛蒡子	Burdock seed
Niuxi	牛膝	Two tooth achyranthes root
Nvzhenzi	女贞子	Glossy privet fruit
	P	
Peilan	佩兰	Fortune eupatorium herb
Pipaye	枇杷叶	Loquat leaf

(Continued)

(Continued)

Chinese Name	中文名	Common Name in English
Pugongying	蒲公英	Dandelion
Puhuang	蒲黄	Cattail pollen
Q		
Qiancao	茜草	India madder root
Qianghuo	羌活	Incised notoptergium rhizome
Qianniuzi	牵牛子	Pharbitis seed
Qianshi	芡实	Gordon euryale seed
Qingdai	青黛	Natural indigo
Qinghao	青蒿	Sweet wormwood herb
Qingpi	青皮	Green tangerine peel
Qinjiao	秦艽	Largeleaf gentian root
Quanxie	全蝎	Scorpion
R		
Rendongteng	忍冬藤	Honeysuckle stem
Renshen	人参	Ginseng
Roucongrong	肉苁蓉	Desertliving cistanche
Rougui	肉桂	Cassia bark
S		
Sangbaipi	桑白皮	White mulberry root-bark
Sangjisheng	桑寄生	Chinese taxillus herb/Mulberry mistletoe stems
Sangshen	桑椹	Mulberry fruit
Sangye	桑叶	Mulberry leaf
Sanleng	三棱	Common burreed tuber
Sanqi	三七	Panax notoginseng
Shanyao	山药	Common yam rhizome
Shanzha	山楂	Hawthorn fruit

(Continued)

(Continued)

Chinese Name	中文名	Common Name in English
Shanzhuyu	山茱萸	Asiatic comelian cherry fruit
Sharen	砂仁	Villous amomum fruit
Shegan	射干	Blackberry lily rhizome
Shejiang	生姜	Fresh ginger
Shengma	升麻	Large trifoliolious bugbane rhizome
Shenjincao	伸筋草	Common club moss
Shichangpu	石菖蒲	Grassleaf sweetflag rhizome
Shigao	石膏	Gypsum
Shihu	石斛	Herba dendrobii
Shijunzi	使君子	Rangooncreeper fruit
Shudihuang	熟地黄	Processed rehmannia root
Shuizhi	水蛭	Leech
Sigua	丝瓜	Loofah
Suanzaoren	酸枣仁	Spine date seed
Sumu	苏木	Sappan wood
Suzi	苏子	Perilla fruit
T		
Taizishen	太子参	Heterophylly false starwort root
Taoren	桃仁	Peach seed
Tianhuafen	天花粉	Snakegourd root
Tianma	天麻	Tall gastrodia tuber
Tinglizi	葶苈子	Pepperweed seed
Tongcao	通草	Ricepaperplant pith
Tufuling	土茯苓	Glabrous greenbrier rhizome
Tusizi	菟丝子	Dodder seed
W		
Wangbuliuxing	王不留行	Cowberb seed
Wugong	蜈蚣	Centipede

(Continued)

(Continued)

Chinese Name	中文名	Common Name in English
Wujiai	五加皮	Slenderstyle acanthopanax bark
Wumei	乌梅	Smoked plum
Wuweizi	五味子	Chinese magnolia vine fruit
Wuyao	乌药	Combined spicebush root
Wuzhuyu	吴茱萸	Medicinal evodia fruit
	X	
Xiakucao	夏枯草	Common selfheal fruit-spike
Xiangfu	香附	Nutgrass galingale rhizome
Xiangru	香薷	Mosia herb
Xianhecao	仙鹤草	Hairyvein agrimonia herb
Xianmao	仙茅	Common curculigo rhizome
Xiebai	薤白	Long-stamen onion bulb
Xinyi	辛夷	Biond magnolia flower
Xixin	细辛	Manchurian wildginger
Xuanfuhua	旋复花	Inula flower
Xuanshen	玄参	Figwort root
Xuchangqing	徐长卿	Paniculate swallowwort root
Xuduan	续断	Himalayan teasel root
Xueyutan	血余炭	Carbonised hair
	Y	
Yanhusuo	延胡索	Rhizoma corydalis/Corydalis tuber
Yejuhua	叶菊花	Wild chrysanthemum flower
Yimucao	益母草	Motherwort herb
Yinchaihu	银柴胡	Starwort root
Yinchen	茵陈	Virgate wormwood herb
Yinyanghuo	淫羊藿	Epimedium herb
Yiyiren	薏苡仁	Coix seeds
Yuanzhi	远志	Thinleaf milkwort root

(Continued)

(Continued)

Chinese Name	中文名	Common Name in English
Yujin	郁金	Tumeric root tuber
Yuxingcao	鱼腥草	Heartleaf houttuynia herb
Yuzhu	玉竹	Fragrant Solomon's seal rhizome
Z		
Zelan	泽兰	Hirsute shiny bugleweed herb
Zexie	泽泻	Oriental waterplantain rhizome
Zhebeimu	浙贝母	Thunberg fritillary bulb
Zhenzhumu	珍珠母	Nacre
Zhifuzi	制附子	Prepared common monkshood daughter root
Zhigancao	炙甘草	Liquorice root processed with honey
Zhimu	知母	Common anemarrhena rhizome
Zhiqiao	枳壳	Orange fruit
Zhishi	枳实	Immature orange fruit
Zhizi	栀子	Cape jasmine fruit
Zhuling	猪苓	Polyporus umbellatus
Zhuru	竹茹	Bamboo shavings
Zicao	紫草	Arnebia root
Zisugeng	紫苏梗	Perilla stem
Zisuye	紫苏叶	Perilla leaf

References

Abrass, IB (1990) The biology and physiology of ageing. *The Western Journal of Medicine*, 153(6): 641-645.

Agus, DB (2012) *The End of Illness*. New York: Free Press.

Atkins, RC (2001) *Dr. Atkins' New Diet Revolution Book*, Revised ed. New York: Avon Books.

Buetter, D (2008) *The Blue Zones*. Washington: National Geographic.

Campbell, TC and Campbell, TM (2004) *The China Study*. Dallas: Benbella Books.

Cheating Death (2016) London: *The Economist*, 13 August, p. 9 and pp. 16-18.

Esselstyn, CB (2008) *Prevent and Reverse Heart Disease*. New York: Avery.

Evans, D (2005) *Placebo: The Belief Effect*. Oxford: Harper Collins.

Hong, H (2016) *Principles of Chinese Medicine: A Modern Interpretation*. London: Imperial College Press.

219

Ilardi, S (2013) Depression as a disease of civilisation, TED talk May 2013. https://www.youtube.com/watch?v=drv3BP0Fdi8 (retrieved 9 September 2016).

Haseeb, J *et al.* (2010) Baseline and on-treatment high-density lipoprotein cholesterol and the risk of cancer in randomized controlled trials of lipid-altering therapy. *Journal of the American College of Cardiology*, 55(25): 2846–2854.

Le Fanu, J (2011) *The Rise and Fall of Modern Medicine*. New York: Hachette Digital.

Needham, J (2016) *Science and Civilisation in China*, Vol VI, Part VI. Cambridge University Press.

New York Times (2015) Nutrition Panel Calls for Less Sugar and Eases Cholesterol and Fat Restrictions. New York: *New York Times*. http://well. blogs.nytimes.com/2015/02/19/nutrition-panel-calls-for-less-sugar-andeases-cholesterol-and-fat-restrictions/ (retrieved 9 September 2016).

Noakes, T (2014) *The Real Meal Revolution*. Cape Town: Quivertree Publications.

Oxford Concise Medical Dictionary (2007) 4th Edition. Oxford: Oxford University Press.

Pollan, M (2006) *The Omnivore's Dilemma*. Penguin.

Rawlins, MD (16 October 2008). *On the Evidence for Decisions About the Use of Therapeutic Interventions*. Harvein Oration, Royal College of Physicians.

Weil, A (1995) *Natural Health, Natural Medicine*. Houghton Mifflin

William Osler Quotes. http://www.brainyquote.com/quotes/authors/w/ william_osler.html (retrieved 8 September 2016).

World Health Organization (2004) *SARS: Clinical Trials on Treatment Using a Combination of Traditional Chinese Medicine and Western Medicine*. http://apps.who.int/medicinedocs/en/d/Js6170e/ (retrieved 8 September, 2016).

World Health Organization (19 August, 2015). *Opening Remarks at the International Forum on Traditional Medicine, China, Macao SAR*. http://who.int/dg/speeches/2015/traditional-medicine/en/ (retrieved 12 September 2016).

Yu, R and Hong, H (2012) *Cancer Management with Chinese Medicine*. Singapore: World Scientific.

《医药六书药性总义》。参考孟仲法著《食疗药膳学》，上海市推卸职工大学教材，1996年八月，177页。

Additional Information on TCM

More information on TCM compiled by the authors may be found on the website of Renhai Corporation Pte Ltd www.renhai.com.sg

The reader may also refer to a number of video presentations by the authors on various aspects of TCM compiled by Council for the 3rd Age (C3A), Singapore:

Videos Titles	Links
The Origins of Chinese Medicine	https://www.youtube.com/watch?v=QhlzCCLSTsU
Methods of TCM	https://www.youtube.com/watch?v=YpWT4ywvLZ4
TCM or Western Medicine?	https://www.youtube.com/watch?v=N8V5-v7TS0U
Deficiency and Tonics	https://www.youtube.com/watch?v=mWBkThGUbWM
Introduction to Qi Tonics	https://www.youtube.com/watch?v=Ey2sOemcBpU
Blood Tonics	https://www.youtube.com/watch?v=Y-ibxlA9NXA
Herbs for Regulating Qi	https://www.youtube.com/watch?v=SeVzIr5ThYE
Herbs for Promoting Digestion	https://www.youtube.com/watch?v=eqiTrR8cBaU
Herbs for Clearing Phlegm & Coughs	https://www.youtube.com/watch?v=CXDvU8iDp2I
Heat clearing Herbs	https://www.youtube.com/watch?v=TXMOCSAq3YQ
Making your Own Herbal Teas Part 1	https://www.youtube.com/watch?v=4Z0i1geGkKY
Making your Own Herbal Teas Part 2	https://www.youtube.com/watch?v=DZL1XLLwcic
Acupressure	https://www.youtube.com/watch?v=FrQOaGnVaWg

Alternatively, the videos may be accessed via the C3A portal: http://www.c3a.org.sg/WatchVideo_process.do?offset=1

Index

Printed in the United States
By Bookmasters